PROFILES OF THE NEWLY LICENSED NURSE:
Historical Trends and Future Implications
Third Edition

Delroy Louden, PhD
Lynda Crawford, PhD, RN
Sherlene Trotman, MS
Division of Research
National League for Nursing

Pub. No. 19-2700

National League for Nursing Press • New York

ISBN 0-88737-660-6

Manufactured in the United States of America

CONTENTS

FOREWORD

This manuscript is the fourth of its kind since the National League for Nursing (NLN) began surveying newly licensed nurses in 1988. At that time, the nursing shortage had led to a demand for reliable nursing work force data. The results of the study were promptly utilized by a wide range of groups from federal, state, and local governments to educators, executives, and policymakers. The Department of Health and Human Services Commission on the Nursing Shortage and the Division of Nursing, have cited this study as an important resource for policy and decision making.

Subsequently, NLN committed to performing the study biennially. Over the past eight years, the data base has grown and expanded our knowledge of the supply and demand for newly registered nurses. More importantly, the data base contains longitudinal data from which historical trends can be traced. In short, the data base on newly licensed nurses is strengthened with each new study.

Much has changed since the first edition of *Profiles of the Newly Licensed Nurse*. As the health care delivery system and economic climate have changed, an increased need for nursing care has been complicated by a decrease in the numbers of nursing positions available. Furthermore, policy initiatives such as health care reform and educational reform will continue to be important contexts that affect the education and employment of registered nurses.

Throughout these turbulent times, executives, educators, recruiters, and government officials look for reliable data on which to base their decisions. We at NLN are ever vigilant to the long-term structural changes in nursing and health care and endeavor to meet these changes in our programs and activities. It is the hope of the researchers at NLN that this volume will contribute valuable information upon which informed changes can occur.

ACKNOWLEDGMENTS

I would like to acknowledge the contribution of everyone without whom this publication would not have been possible. First and foremost, Donna Post, PhD, Research Coordinator, who provided invaluable assistance in analyzing the mammoth data base on newly licensed nurses. Her methodical and patient approach to research facilitated the smooth progression of steps to the completion of the study.

Secondly, I'd like to recognize the 1994 cohort of newly licensed registered nurses for responding to our survey and helping us better understand the labor issues surrounding our newest entrant to the nursing supply. As a group, they display an unusually high level of commitment to the profession and to health care. They are to be commended and respected for their contribution to the common good.

NEWLY LICENSED NURSES SURVEY: AN OVERVIEW

In 1988, the National League for Nursing (NLN) surveyed newly licensed nurses in response to an unprecedented demand for data about nursing resources. The demand had been created by a nursing shortage; hospitals were unable to fill nursing positions, and nursing school enrollments were declining. The survey provided information that was useful to employers and educators alike during the most critical period of shortages.

[1]Since the initial 1988 survey, NLN has continued to collect information about newly licensed nurses every two years. Trends have been noted regarding graduates' demographics, education enrollments, and employment opportunities. Many trends have reflected the changing health care environment, as well as changes in the nursing work force.

Information on nurses continues to be in demand. Nurses comprise the largest group of health care providers and, as such, will make a significant impact on the delivery of health care in the future. As models of health care delivery in this country continue to change, agencies and facilities are concerned with the efficient utilization of nurses. Schools of

Note: References appear on p. 119.

1

nursing are interested in reaching potential students more efficiently.

RESEARCH DESIGN AND METHODOLOGY

The purpose of this study was to collect information regarding the demographics, education, and employment status of newly licensed nurses in the United States. The questions asked were consistent with those of the previous surveys so that patterns across time can be discerned.

Surveys were mailed to all individuals who received their formal nursing education in the United States and had successfully completed their licensing examinations in the month of July 1993. All newly licensed nurses were sent a copy of the survey to be completed. Names and addresses of respondents were obtained from the National Council of State Boards of Nursing, the examining body of the NCLEX-RN exam. Prior approval was granted from all state boards of nursing except those of New Hampshire and Hawaii, which do not allow the release of such information.

The survey tool contained 29 questions covering (a) demographic characteristics, (b) educational situations, (c) employment status, (d) types of employers, and (e) perception of education (Figure 1.1). A space for comments was included.

The surveys were personalized with precoded information regarding school code, state, and program type. They were machine readable of the type commonly used in national standardized examinations.

In an effort to achieve a high response rate, a series of three mailings with telephone follow-ups were completed. The 1994 response rate (64.8%) was higher than in 1992 (63.5%) but varied considerably from state to state (Table 1.1). The state with the highest response rate was Wisconsin (76.5%), followed by Minnesota (74.4%), Montana (74.25%), and Wyoming (73.3%). Mississippi had the lowest (56.5%).

This preliminary chapter will be followed by detailed information of the survey results. All data is correlated with key variables such as program type, geographic region, and trends from previous years. Results are illustrated in the figures and tables throughout the book. Data from each of nine census regions are separated to provide information on geographic differences where useful (Figure 1.2). Data from individual states are provided whenever possible.

In Chapter 2, the demographic profiles of the new nurses are described. Age, racial/ethnic background, residency, marital status, presence of children in the home, and previous education and experience are presented. Due to the low response rate from minorities and men, data presented will be limited to information on enrollment by type of program.

The educational experiences of newly licensed nurses is presented in Chapter 3, including the evaluation by respondents of their classroom and clinical experiences. In addition, data regarding previous experience as LPN/LVNs, prior education, and participation in an NCLEX-RN review course are also included.

The primary focus of Chapter 4 is on employment status. Data presented include employment settings, the length of time it took to find jobs, respondents' perceptions of job availability, the reasons they selected their current positions, and information regarding salaries. Data obtained from the 1994 survey are contrasted with 1992 data.

A profile of newly licensed practical/vocational nurses is the primary focus of Chapter 5. This information is included for the first time in the history of the publication. The survey was initiated in 1994 by the National Council of State Boards of Nursing and includes demographic, education, and employment characteristics of LPN/LVNs licensed in 1993.

Chapter 6 is a summary of the preceding text discussing the comments and concerns of survey participants. Several distinct themes emerge from the data regarding employment experiences of new graduates and the availability of jobs.

This book is a report on feedback from a group of new nurses from across the country. Their message is relevant for everyone concerned with the health of the nation.

Figure 1.1 Survey Sample

EMPLOYMENT OF NEWLY LICENSED NURSES

Mark Reflex® by NCS EM-40243/321 Printed in U.S.A.

National League for Nursing
350 Hudson Street
New York, New York 10014

DIRECTIONS FOR MARKING QUESTIONNAIRE SHEET
Use Black lead pencil only (No. 2)
Do NOT use ink or ballpoint pens
Make heavy black marks that fill oval completely
Erase cleanly any answer you wish to change
MAKE NO MARKS IN SHADED AREAS

Examples of IMPROPER marks   Examples of PROPER marks

PLEASE MAKE ANY NECESSARY CHANGES TO NAME AND ADDRESS   MARK IF ANY CHANGE →

PLEASE NOTE: ALL INFORMATION ON THIS FORM WILL BE HELD IN THE STRICTEST CONFIDENCE.
NO INDIVIDUAL'S RESPONSES WILL BE RELEASED OR REPORTED.

1 Year of Graduation → 19

2 Did you attend nursing school
- ○ Full time?
- ○ Part time?

3 Did you take an NCLEX-RN review course?
- ○ Yes
- ○ No

4 Did you hold an LPN/LVN before starting your RN education?
- ○ Yes
- ○ No

4a How long did you work as a LPN/LVN before becoming a RN?
- ○ never
- ○ less than 1 year
- ○ 1 – 3 years
- ○ 3 – 5 years
- ○ over 5 years

5 Mark one statement that most nearly corresponds to your most recent job-hunting experiences in nursing:
- ○ Many jobs were available
- ○ A fair number of jobs were available
- ○ Very few jobs were available
- ○ Can't say — took job at clinical site
- ○ Can't say — voluntarily unemployed

COMPLETE EITHER Q. 6, 7 OR 8 TO BEST DESCRIBE YOUR CURRENT EMPLOYMENT SITUATION

6 ○ I am employed in nursing — not seeking another job

CONTINUE TO QUESTION **9**

7 I am employed in nursing —
- ○ but seeking other job in nursing
- ○ but seeking other job not in nursing

Which of the following incentives would MOST convince you to stay at your current job? (Mark one?)
- ○ Better salary/benefits
- ○ Flexible/better schedule or hours
- ○ Change clinical area
- ○ Opportunity for career advancement
- ○ Better staffing/working conditions
- ○ Other (explain below)
- ○ Nothing could keep me (explain below)

Explain:

CONTINUE TO QUESTION **9**

8 ○ I am employed, not in nursing, but am seeking a job in nursing
○ I am employed, not in nursing, and am not seeking a job in nursing
○ I am presently not employed

Main reason why not employed in nursing (Mark one):
- ○ No jobs
- ○ Jobs available, but couldn't find what I wanted
- ○ Continuing my education
- ○ Family responsibilities
- ○ Have relocated
- ○ Don't want to practice nursing
- ○ Other:

→ How long have you been actively seeking a nursing job?
- ○ One month or less
- ○ Two to three months
- ○ Four to six months
- ○ Over six months
- ○ Not seeking a job

PLEASE SKIP TO QUESTION **20**

9 Since receiving your RN license, is this your
- ○ 1st
- ○ 2nd
- ○ 3rd or more job in nursing?

10 How long after graduation did it take you to find your first job in nursing? (Mark one):
- ○ Found the job before graduation
- ○ One month or less
- ○ Two to three months
- ○ Four to six months
- ○ Over six months

11 How did you find out about your current job? (Mark one):
- ○ Classified ad in newspaper/journal
- ○ Word-of-mouth
- ○ Faculty recommendation
- ○ Clinical site for nursing school
- ○ On-site recruiter
- ○ Employment agency
- ○ Other:

12 Mark the two main reasons for choosing your current position:
- ○ Amount of vacation/holidays
- ○ Housing
- ○ Health insurance
- ○ Tuition reimbursement
- ○ Salary/benefits
- ○ Promotional opportunities
- ○ Had externship there
- ○ Desired this specialization
- ○ Other:

13 Employment Status in nursing:
- ○ Full time
- ○ Part time — less than 20 hours/week
- ○ Part time — 20 or more hours/week
- ○ Work as needed/ per diem

14 Type of position:
- ○ General duty/staff
- ○ Head nurse/assistant
- ○ Private duty
- ○ Other:

PLEASE CONTINUE TO QUESTION **15** ON REVERSE SIDE

5

Figure 1.1 (continued)

15 Type of employer (Mark one):

- ○ Hospital
- ○ Nursing Home
- ○ Comm., Home or Public Health Agency
- ○ Temporary Agency
- ○ School Nurse/Physician's Office
- ○ Other

15a HOSPITAL UNIT:
Which unit do you primarily work in? (Mark one):

- ○ Medical/Surgical
- ○ Critical care (any type)
- ○ Operating room
- ○ Obstetrics/Gyn
- ○ Emergency room
- ○ Outpatient department
- ○ Pediatrics
- ○ Other:

16 Please specify the annual earnings from your primary nursing position before tax deductions. Do NOT include overtime.

17 How well did your classroom and clinical experiences prepare you for your current job?

Classroom	Clinical
○ Excellent	○ Excellent
○ Very good	○ Very good
○ Good	○ Good
○ Fair	○ Fair
○ Poor	○ Poor

If you rated your clinical experiences fair or poor, what was the primary reason?

- ○ Disorganized/fragmented use of time
- ○ Insufficient time
- ○ Insufficient exposure to technology
- ○ Poor faculty
- ○ Poor facilities
- ○ Other:

18 Are you represented by a labor association that has a contract for collective bargaining?

- ○ Yes
- ○ No
- ○ Don't Know

19 My work orientation was:

- ○ Excellent
- ○ Very good
- ○ Good
- ○ Fair
- ○ Poor

20 Did you have a college degree before going to nursing school?

- ○ Yes
- ○ No

If yes, what was your highest earned credential?

- ○ Associate Degree
- ○ Bachelor's Degree
- ○ Master's Degree
- ○ Doctoral Degree

21 If you had a college degree, what was your major field of study?

- ○ Health related
- ○ Biological or physical science
- ○ Business or management
- ○ Education
- ○ Liberal Arts
- ○ Social science
- ○ Other:

22 Sex:
- ○ Female
- ○ Male

23 Racial/Ethnic background:
- ○ White (Non-hispanic)
- ○ Black (Non-hispanic)
- ○ Hispanic
- ○ Asian American
- ○ American Indian

24 Year of Birth
19___

25 Marital status:
- ○ Never married
- ○ Married
- ○ Separated/Divorced
- ○ Widowed

26 Children living at home most of the time are: (Mark one):
- ○ No children at home
- ○ All less than 6 years old
- ○ All 6 years old or older
- ○ Both younger and older than 6 years

27 Residency immediately before attending nursing school:

STATE

COUNTY

ZIP CODE

28 Residency immediately after graduating from nursing school:

STATE

COUNTY

ZIP CODE

29 Location of current place of employment:

STATE

COUNTY

ZIP CODE

COMMENTS:

THANK YOU FOR YOUR TIME AND COOPERATION. YOUR PARTICIPATION IN THIS SURVEY WILL GREATLY BENEFIT THE NURSING COMMUNITY.
PLEASE RETURN THE COMPLETED QUESTIONNAIRE AS SOON AS POSSIBLE IN THE ENCLOSED POSTAGE-PAID ENVELOPE.

Figure 1.2 Census Regions of the United States

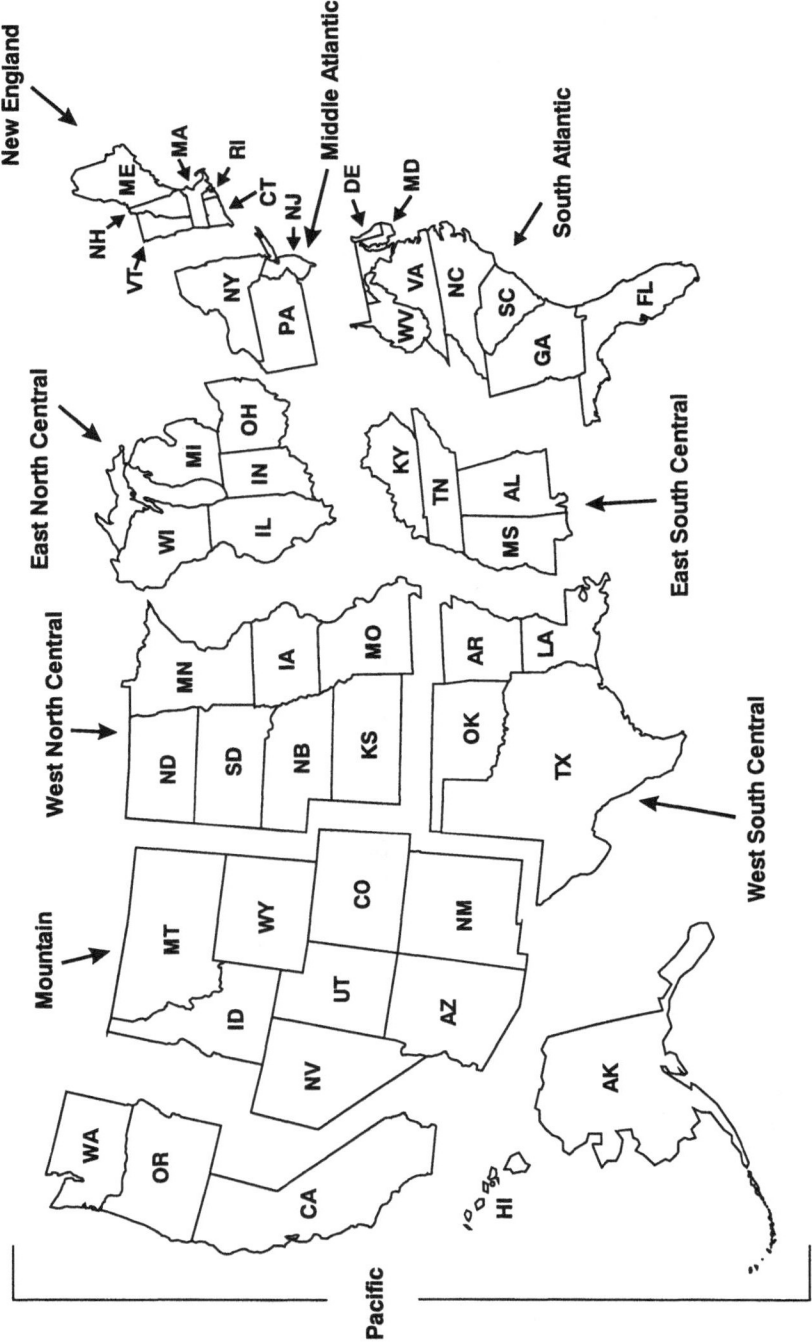

Table 1.1   Response Rate by State in which Attended Nursing School, Newly Licensed Nurses, 1994

STATE*	NUMBER OF RESPONDENTS	RESPONSE RATE
Alabama	757	58.68
Alaska	35	66.04
Arizona	380	62.60
Arkansas	454	62.11
California	2,125	64.20
Colorado	486	67.03
Connecticut	498	66.40
Delaware	129	64.82
District of Columbia	30	57.69
Florida	1,565	62.43
Georgia	1,143	62.32
Idaho	184	71.88
Illinois	1,787	61.26
Indiana	1,097	68.95
Iowa	686	68.06
Kansas	581	65.80
Kentucky	926	63.21
Louisiana	644	64.46
Maine	251	70.11
Maryland	741	66.64
Massachusetts	1,202	64.31
Michigan	1,361	64.90
Minnesota	965	74.46
Mississippi	554	56.53
Missouri	966	63.64
Montana	124	74.25
Nebraska	344	69.08
Nevada	112	72.73
New Jersey	1,174	66.07
New Mexico	189	66.08
New York	2,452	59.03
North Carolina	1,320	59.89
North Dakota	147	69.67
Ohio	2,191	67.92
Oklahoma	616	60.10
Oregon	489	68.97

(continued)

Table 1.1   Response Rate by State in which Attended Nursing School, Newly Licensed Nurses, 1994 (continued)

STATE*	NUMBER OF RESPONDENTS	RESPONSE RATE
Pennsylvania	2,936	71.77
Rhode Island	202	66.01
South Carolina	535	68.68
South Dakota	200	64.72
Tennessee	1,008	61.88
Texas	2,423	62.34
Utah	317	68.76
Vermont	102	68.46
Virginia	1,009	64.93
Washington	634	66.32
West Virginia	427	64.60
Wisconsin	859	76.49
Wyoming	162	73.30
Unknown	13	56.52
TOTAL	39,584	64.84

*   The State Boards of Nursing in Hawaii and New Hampshire have refused permission to release information on their new licensees despite several attempts to persuade them otherwise. Since these states have relatively small representation, their absence will not prejudice the findings of this study. Due to mail forwarding, some newly licensed nurses from these two states received and responded to the survey. However, these respondents cannot be considered representative of these states.

CHARACTERISTICS OF THE NEWLY LICENSED NURSE

2

This chapter will provide an overview of the demographic characteristics of the 1994 newly licensed nurse.

The numbers of newly licensed nurses by region and state are listed in Table 3.3. The East North Central region reported the most newly licensed nurses (7,297) and includes the states of Illinois, Indiana, Michigan, Ohio, and Wisconsin. The region with the least number of new nurses (1,954) includes states such as Arizona, Colorado, Idaho, and Montana. The state with the most nurses continues to be Pennsylvania (2,936), followed by New York (2,453) and Texas (2,423). The states with the least numbers of new nurses were Hawaii (9), the District of Columbia (30), and Alaska (35).

AGE

The average age of newly licensed nurses has shown a slight decline in general (Figure 2.1). This is a reverse in the trend that was noted in 1992, when the average age of newly licensed nurses was on the rise. The mean age across all program types was 31.5, compared with 32.1 in 1992.

Differences in age among program types have remained consistent.

Most respondents (56.3%) were 33 years of age or younger (Table 2.1). Although 20.4 % were between the ages of 22 to 24, 22.9% were over the age of 40. Diploma and baccalaureate graduates were younger overall than associate degree graduates.

MARITAL STATUS

The number of newly licensed nurses who were married or separated/divorced has continued to increase since 1990 (Figure 2.2) while the number who were widowed remained the same. More than half of the respondents were married. By program type, most (64.5%) associate degree graduates were married, compared to half (50.1%) of the diploma and less than half (44.1%) of the baccalaureate graduates (Figure 2.3). A greater proportion of baccalaureate graduates had never been married. Among associate degree nurses, a greater proportion (16.0%) were separated or divorced than those from the other two types of programs.

Between 1992 and 1994, there was little difference in the number of respondents with children in the home (Figure 2.5). A greater proportion (45.4%) of diploma graduates had children in the home while baccalaureate students had the smallest proportion (28.9%).

MINORITY AND MALE STUDENTS

While most nurses are white females, a greater proportion of minority students graduated from nursing programs in 1994 than in 1992 (Figure 2.6). Respondents were identified as either white (non-Hispanic), black (non-Hispanic), Hispanic, Asian American, or American Indian. Minority representation was highest among those identified as black (6.8%) and lowest among American Indians (0.6%) (Table 2.2). There has been a gradual decline in the proportion of black graduates since 1990 and a gradual increase in Asian graduates (Figure 2.6). The proportions of Hispanic and American Indian groups have remained consistent.

The number of men who graduated from basic RN programs has increased since 1992, representing 11.4 percent of the 1994 respondents (Figure 2.7). The proportion of men in each type of program was similar (Table 2.2).

Figure 2.1   Average Age of Newly Licensed Nurses By Program Type, 1990, 1992, 1994

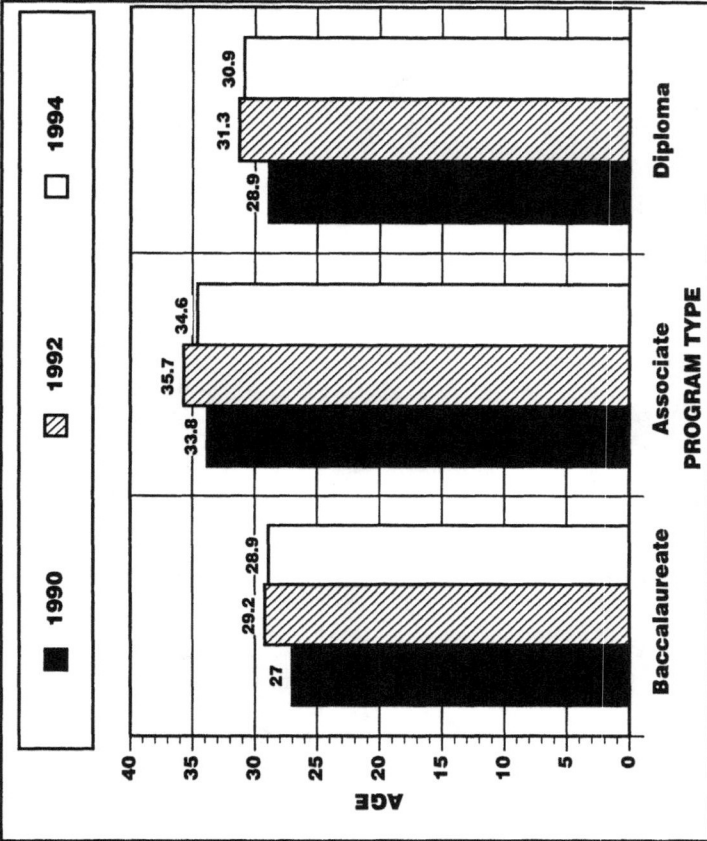

Figure 2.2 Marital Status of Newly Licensed Nurses, 1990, 1992, 1994

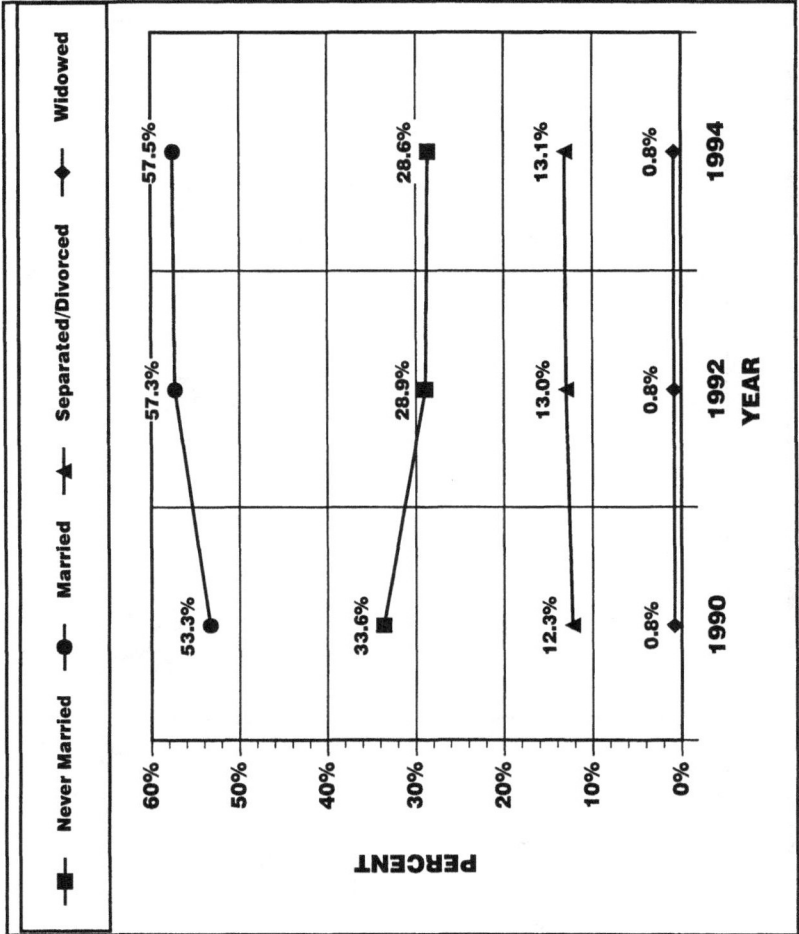

Figure 2.3 Marital Status of Newly Licensed Nurses by Program Type, 1994

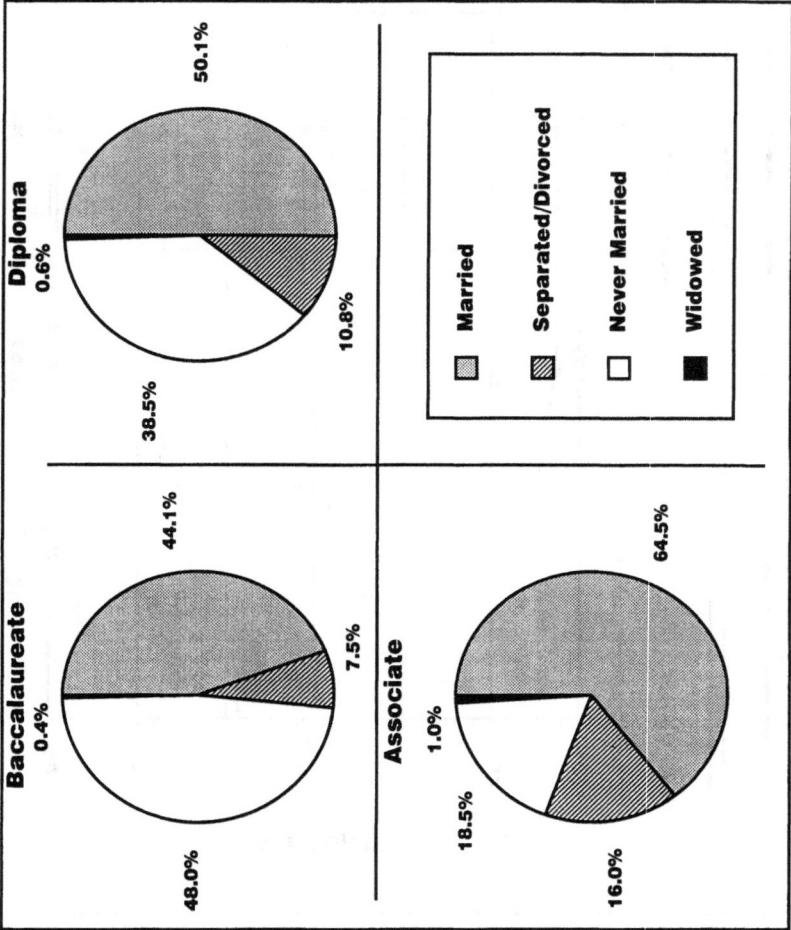

Baccalaureate

- 0.4%
- 44.1%
- 7.5%
- 48.0%

Diploma

- 0.6%
- 50.1%
- 10.8%
- 38.5%

Associate

- 1.0%
- 64.5%
- 16.0%
- 18.5%

Legend:
- ▨ Married
- ▨ Separated/Divorced
- ☐ Never Married
- ■ Widowed

16

Figure 2.4   Presence of Children at Home by Program Type, 1994

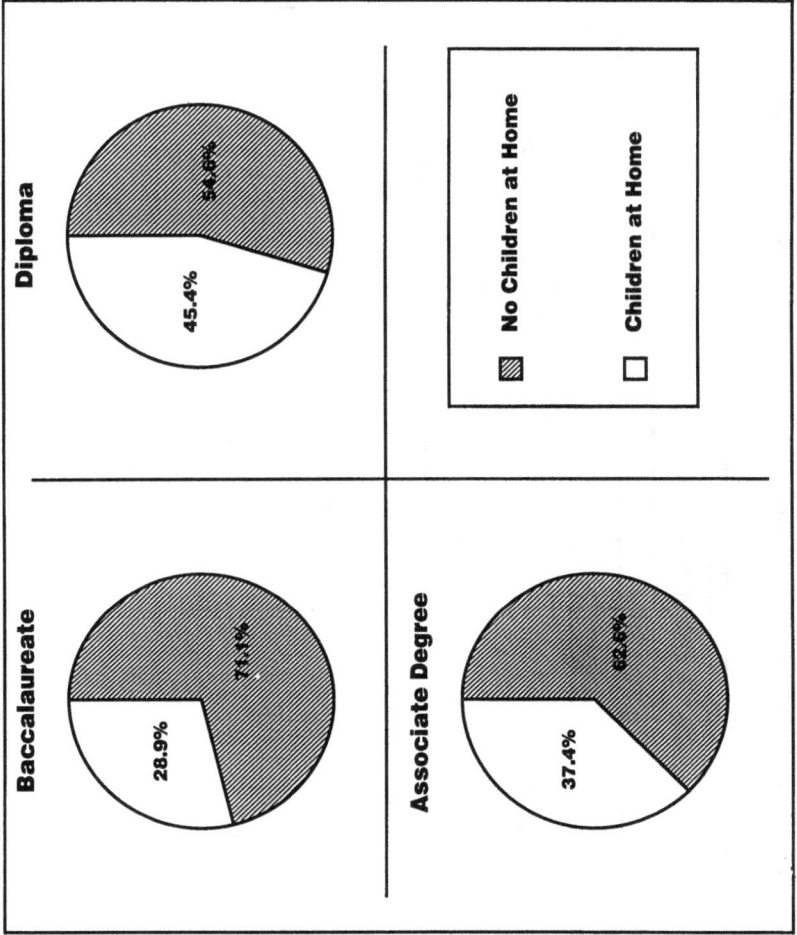

Diploma

45.4% 54.6%

Baccalaureate

28.9% 71.1%

Associate Degree

37.4% 62.6%

▨ No Children at Home

☐ Children at Home

Figure 2.5   Presence of Children at Home, 1990, 1992, 1994

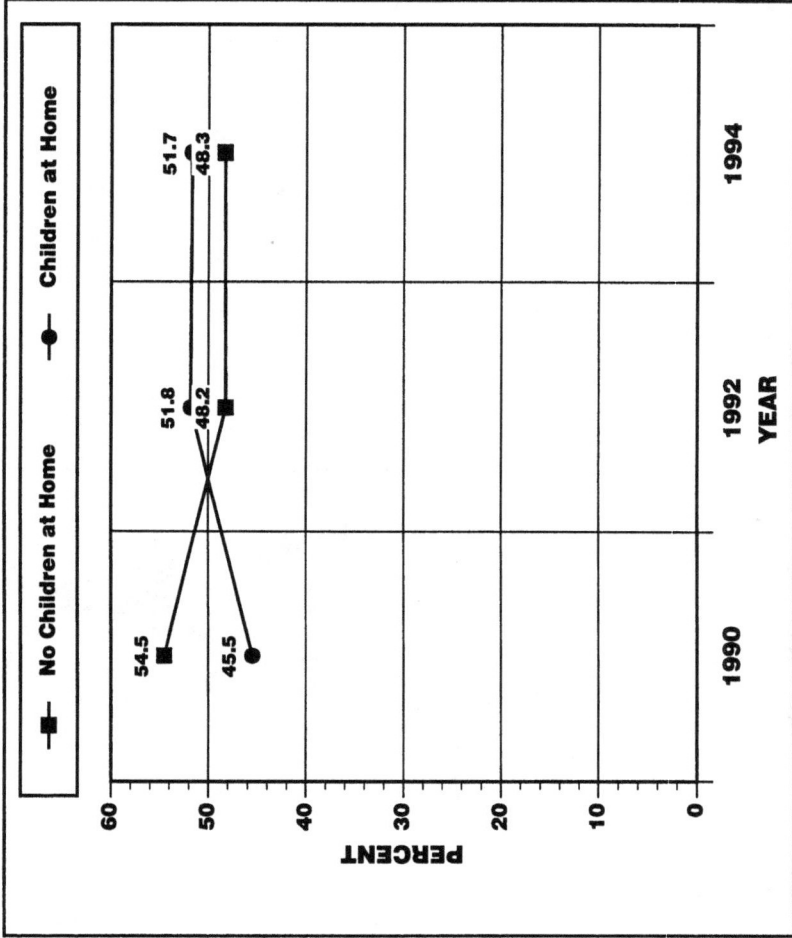

Legend: ■ No Children at Home   ● Children at Home

	1990	1992	1994
No Children at Home	54.5	48.2	48.3
Children at Home	45.5	51.8	51.7

PERCENT (y-axis: 0, 10, 20, 30, 40, 50, 60)

YEAR (x-axis)

Figure 2.6   Proportion of Minority Students Graduating from Basic RN Programs, 1990, 1992, 1994

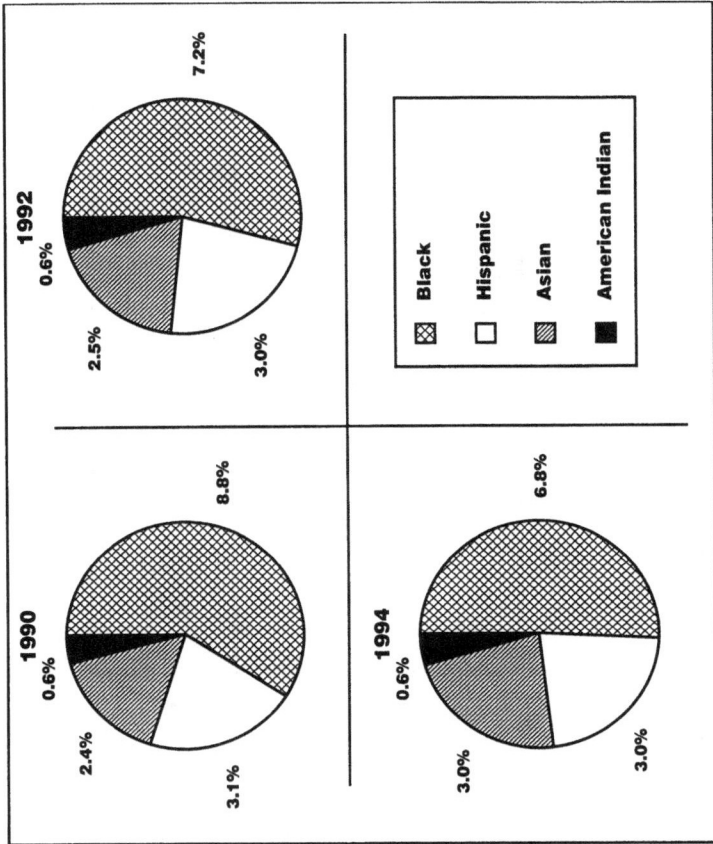

Source: Nursing DataSource 1995, Volume I.

Figure 2.7   Percentage of Men Who Graduated from Basic RN Programs, 1991, 1992, 1993, 1994

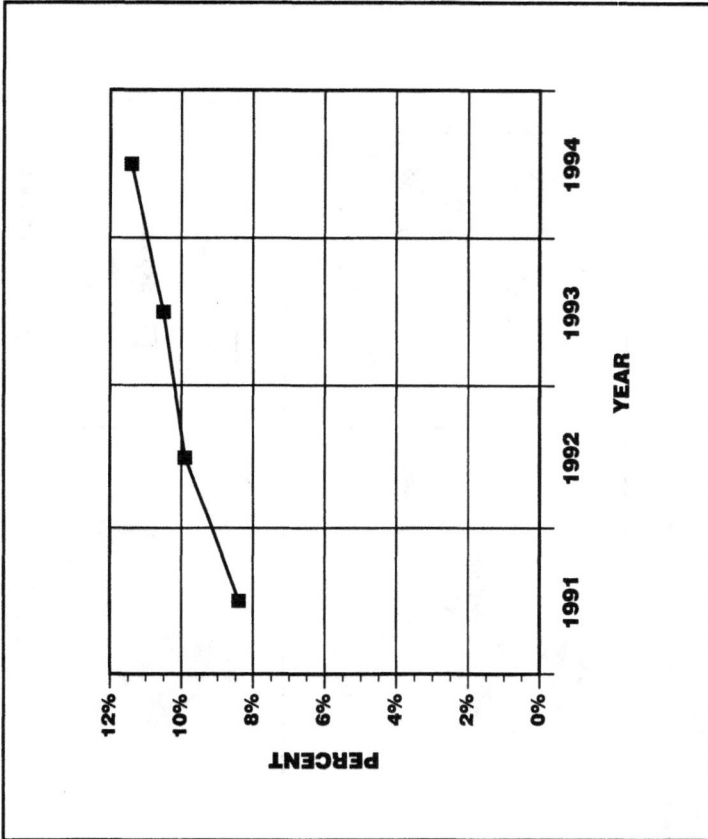

Source: *Nursing DataSource 1995, Volume I.*

Table 2.1 Demographic Profile of Newly Licensed Nurses

| | | | | | PROGRAM TYPE | | | |
| | TOTAL | | Diploma | | Associate Degree | | Baccalaureate | |
	Number	Percent	Number	Percent	Number	Percent	Number	Percent
TOTAL	37,262	100.0	2,962	100.0	23,758	100.0	10,542	100.0
AGE								
21 or Younger	369	1.0	71	2.4	297	1.3	1	0.0
22-24	7,618	20.4	746	25.2	2,570	10.8	4,302	40.8
25-27	4,942	13.3	498	16.8	2,400	10.1	2,044	19.4
28-30	3,977	10.7	325	11.0	2,679	11.3	973	9.2
31-33	4,078	10.9	317	10.7	2,952	12.4	809	7.7
34-36	3,947	10.6	248	8.4	3,060	12.9	639	6.1
37-39	3,826	10.3	262	8.8	2,967	12.5	597	5.7
40-42	3,203	8.6	199	6.7	2,527	10.6	477	4.5
43-55	5,090	13.7	281	9.5	4,129	17.4	680	6.5
56 or Older	212	0.6	15	0.5	177	0.7	20	0.2

(continued)

Table 2.1 (continued)

	TOTAL		PROGRAM TYPE							
			Diploma		Associate Degree		Baccalaureate			
	Number	Percent	Number	Percent	Number	Percent	Number	Percent		

MARITAL STATUS

	TOTAL Number	TOTAL Percent	Diploma Number	Diploma Percent	Associate Degree Number	Associate Degree Percent	Baccalaureate Number	Baccalaureate Percent
TOTAL	**35,345**	**100.0**	**2,807**	**100.0**	**22,352**	**100.0**	**10,186**	**100.0**
Never Married	10,106	28.6	1,080	38.5	4,132	18.5	4,894	48.0
Married	20,320	57.5	1,406	50.1	14,423	64.5	4,491	44.1
Separated/Divorced	4,641	13.1	304	10.8	3,574	16.0	763	7.5
Widowed	278	.8	17	.6	223	1.0	38	.4

PRESENCE OF CHILDREN

TOTAL	**34,124**	**100.0**	**2,669**	**100.0**	**21,773**	**100.0**	**9,682**	**100.0**
No Children at Home	16,479	48.3	1,456	54.6	8,137	37.4	6,886	71.1
Has Children at Home	17,645	51.7	1,213	45.4	13,636	62.6	2,796	28.9

22

Table 2.2 Demographic Profile of Students Graduating from Basic RN Programs, by Program Type, 1994

			PROGRAM TYPE					
	TOTAL		Diploma		Associate Degree		Baccalaureate	
	Number	Percent	Number	Percent	Number	Percent	Number	Percent
RACIAL/ETHNIC BACKGROUND								
TOTAL	**94,870**	**100.0**	**7,119**	**100.0**	**58,839**	**100.0**	**28,912**	**100.0**
White[1]	81,449	85.9	6,280	88.2	50,602	86.0	24,567	85.0
Black[1]	6,455	6.8	393	5.5	4,150	7.1	1,912	6.6
Hispanic[1]	2,841	3.0	181	2.5	1,790	3.0	870	3.0
Asian[1]	2,796	3.0	205	2.9	1,475	2.5	1,116	3.9
American Indian[1]	566	0.6	24	0.4	409	0.7	133	0.5
Other/Unknown[1]	726	0.7	34	0.5	385	0.7	307	1.0
GENDER								
TOTAL	**79,953**	**100.0**	**6,733**	**100.0**	**47,870**	**100.0**	**25,350**	**100.0**
Female	70,823	88.6	5,928	88.0	42,361	88.5	22,534	88.9
Male	9,130	11.4	805	12.0	5,509	11.5	2,816	11.1

[1]Based on estimations. Due to rounding, the estimations sometimes add up to slightly less than the true total.

EDUCATIONAL PROFILE

3

*"I'm not disappointed in my classroom educa-
tion. However, I feel my clinical experiences and
learning were limited. Therefore, after graduation,
I had the book knowledge but lacked the hands-
on skill I felt was expected of me by my employer.
This is an area I feel needs changing in nursing."*
(Tennessee)

Respondents answered questions regarding activity levels
while they were students, prior experiences and education,
the adequacy of their education, and participation in NCLEX
review courses. Respondents across all program types wrote
additional comments regarding their educational experiences
on the survey form.

TYPES OF PROGRAMS ATTENDED

Table 3.2 lists the 1,501 basic RN programs by region and
state. The region with the most programs continues to be the
East North Central (267 programs) and includes such states as
Illinois and Ohio. New York is the state with the most (100)
programs; Alaska has the fewest (2).

Since 1988, there has been a dramatic shift in nursing
education away from the hospital-based diploma program
toward college-based associate and baccalaureate programs.
In 1994, the numbers of associate and baccalaureate programs continued to rise steadily, while the number of di-

ploma programs was declining (Figure 3.2). Over half of all RN programs were associate degree programs.

More than two-thirds of newly licensed nurses responding to the survey held associate degrees (Table 3.1), which was representative of the total population of graduates (Table 6.1). The largest increase in percent of graduates by program type was in baccalaureate programs.

ACTIVITY LEVELS

An overwhelming majority of the respondents had attended school full-time (Figure 3.1). Baccalaureate degree respondents reported the highest percentage of full-time attendance at 96 percent while diploma programs had the largest percentage of part-time students. The number of students attending nursing school full-time increased slightly in 1994 for baccalaureate and associate degree programs but decreased for diploma programs.

PRIOR EXPERIENCE

Licensed practical nurses/licensed vocational nurses (LPN/LVN) appear to be an excellent group of individuals to seek as potential applicants for basic RN programs. They are generally adult learners who see the need during their professional experience to expand their careers, gaining more responsibility and opportunity for advancement. RN programs provide education that builds upon their knowledge and experience. Most LPN/LVNs who graduated from nursing school in 1994 attended associate degree programs (Figure 3.3). Baccalaureate schools had attracted the fewest LPN/LVN students.

Of those who worked as LPN/LVNs, half had worked more than five years (Figure 3.4). Approximately 16 percent had worked one to three years. It is interesting that more than eight percent having LPN/LVN licensure had never worked as LPN/LVNs. Fewer nurses holding associate degrees and licensed in 1994 (24.4. %) had worked as LPN/LVNs than those licensed in 1992 (32.1%). The same was true for all other program types.

26

PRIOR EDUCATION

Individuals with prior college degrees are also an excellent group of potential applicants for RN programs. Nursing appears to be an attractive discipline for individuals considering returning to college to continue their education or for those seeking career changes. More than 22 percent of the 1994 respondents held college degrees prior to attending nursing school (Figure 3.5). While these nurses held degrees ranging from the associate to the doctoral levels, slightly more than half of them held baccalaureate degrees (Table 3.4).

Returning students held degrees in various fields of study, most frequently liberal arts and health-related fields (Figure 3.6). Although most of these returning students enrolled in baccalaureate degree nursing programs, those holding associate degrees tended to enter associate degree programs (Table 3.4).

ADEQUACY OF EDUCATION

Respondents were asked to assess the adequacy of their classroom and clinical experiences in preparing them for their current jobs. This feedback is valuable for increasing our awareness of the deficiencies in nursing education. Most respondents rated their classroom and clinical experiences as adequate, responding either "excellent," "very good," or "good." (Responses of "fair" or "poor" were consolidated as "not adequate" ratings.) Ratings were higher than those of the 1992 survey (Figure 3.7).

There were differences in the level of satisfaction students felt by program type (Table 3.5). Diploma graduates rated their classroom and clinical experiences substantially higher than associate and baccalaureate degree nurses. Diploma graduates tended to give the highest overall ratings and associate degree graduates the lowest.

There were several reasons cited for inadequate clinical experiences (Figure 3.8). The most commonly reported reasons were those of insufficient time and insufficient exposure to technology. Other reasons included disorganized/fragmented use of time, poor facilities, and poor faculty. Insufficient time was also the primary reason for fair or poor ratings of clinical experience by program type (Table 3.6).

PARTICIPATION IN NCLEX-RN REVIEW COURSE

Most newly licensed nurses had elected to take the NCLEX-RN review course (Figure 3.9). A higher percentage of baccalaureate students took this course than associate degree and diploma counterparts. More individuals elected to take the review course in 1994 than in 1992.

Figure 3.1   Nursing School Attendance by Program Type, 1994

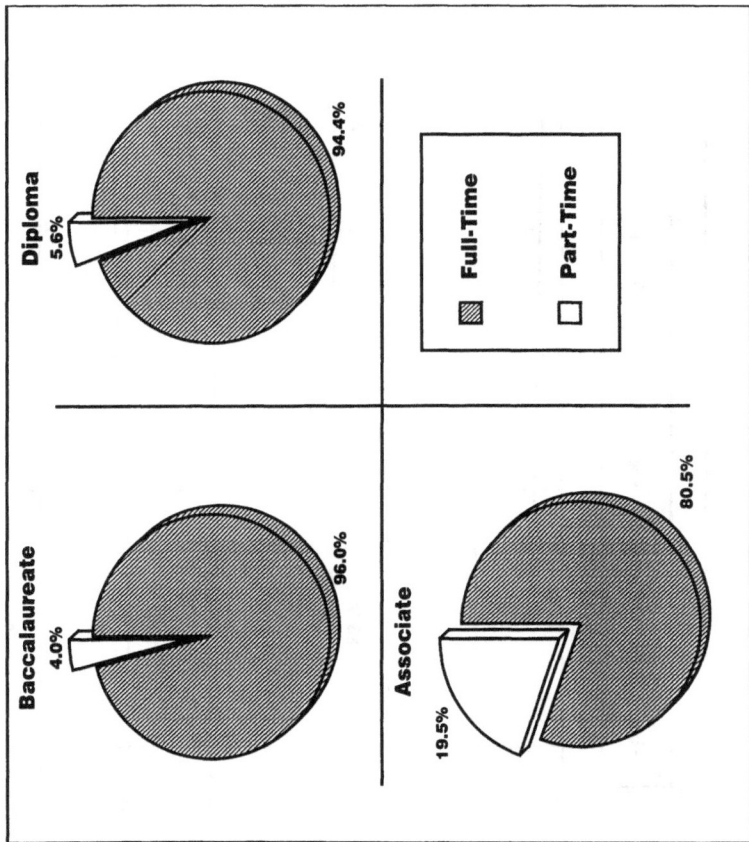

Baccalaureate

4.0%   96.0%

Diploma

5.6%   94.4%

Associate

19.5%   80.5%

Full-Time

Part-Time

Figure 3.2 Proportion of Basic RN Programs by Program Type, 1990, 1992, 1994

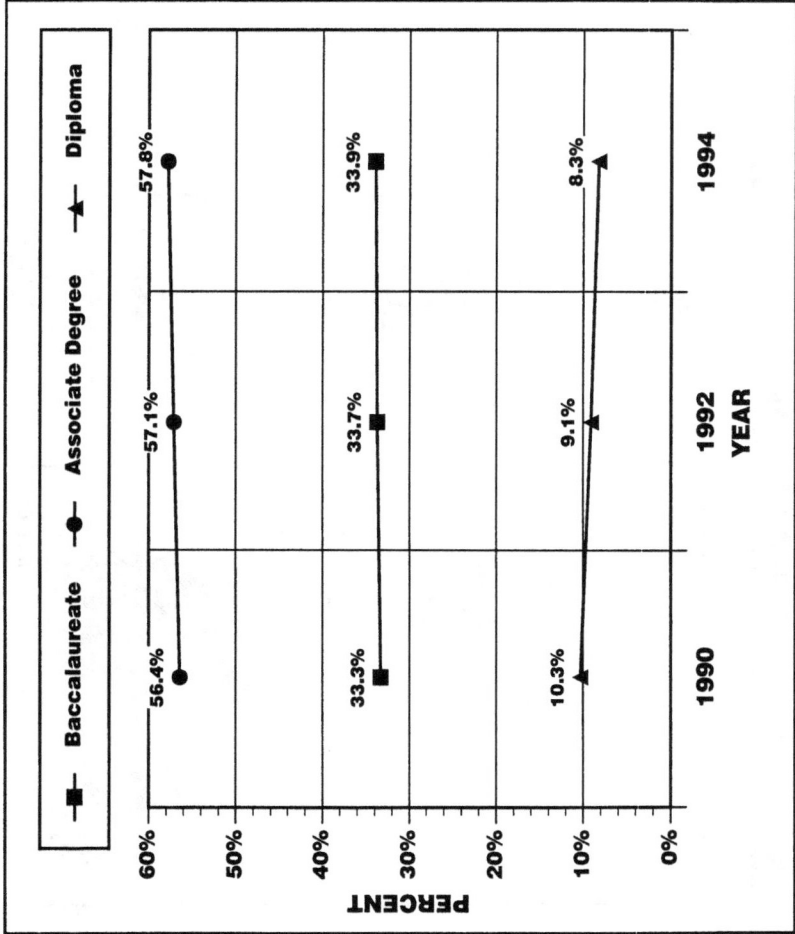

Legend:
- Baccalaureate
- Associate Degree
- Diploma

Program Type	1990	1992	1994
Baccalaureate	56.4%	57.1%	57.8%
Associate Degree	33.3%	33.7%	33.9%
Diploma	10.3%	9.1%	8.3%

PERCENT (y-axis: 0% – 60%)

YEAR (x-axis)

Figure 3.3   Newly Licensed Nurses with Prior LPN/LVN License by Program Type, 1994

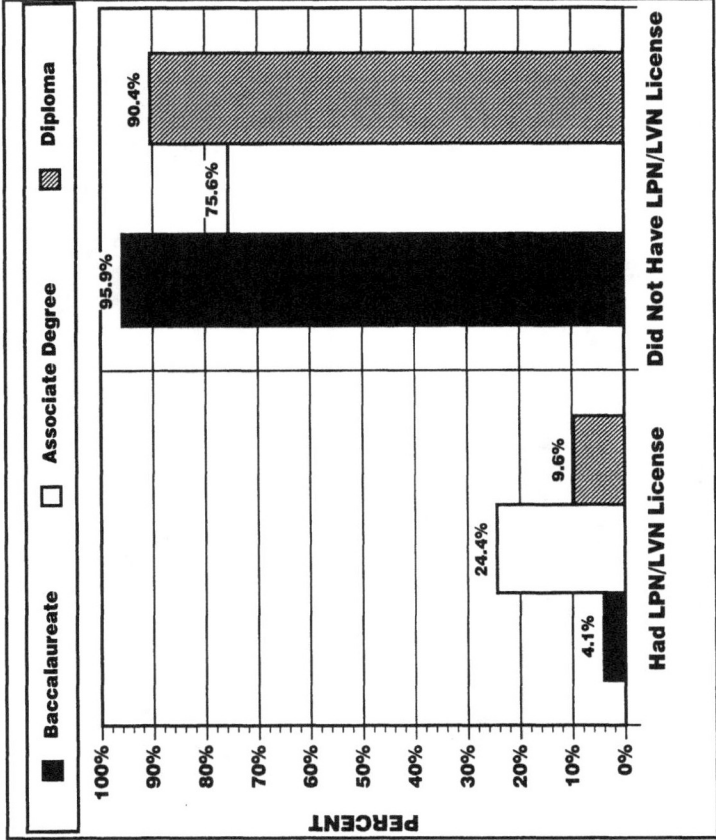

Figure 3.4   Length of Time Newly Licensed Nurses Worked as LPN/LVN, 1994

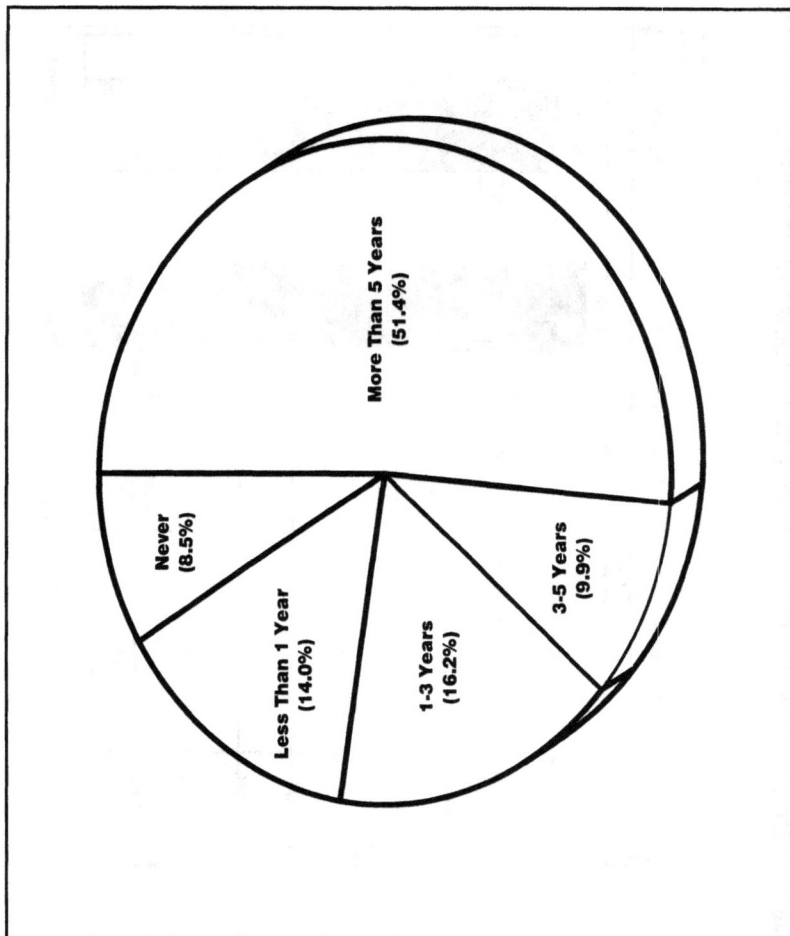

Never
(8.5%)

Less Than 1 Year
(14.0%)

1-3 Years
(16.2%)

3-5 Years
(9.9%)

More Than 5 Years
(51.4%)

Figure 3.5   Newly Licensed Nurses Who Held a College Degree Prior to Attending Nursing School, by Program Type, 1994

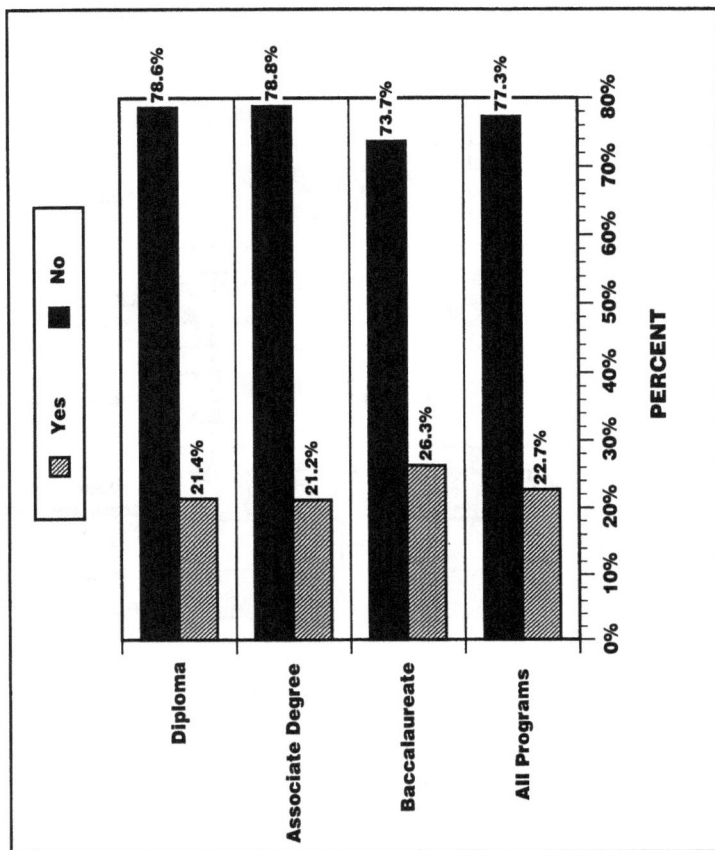

33

Figure 3.6   Major Field of Study of Newly Licensed Nurses with Previous College Degree, 1994

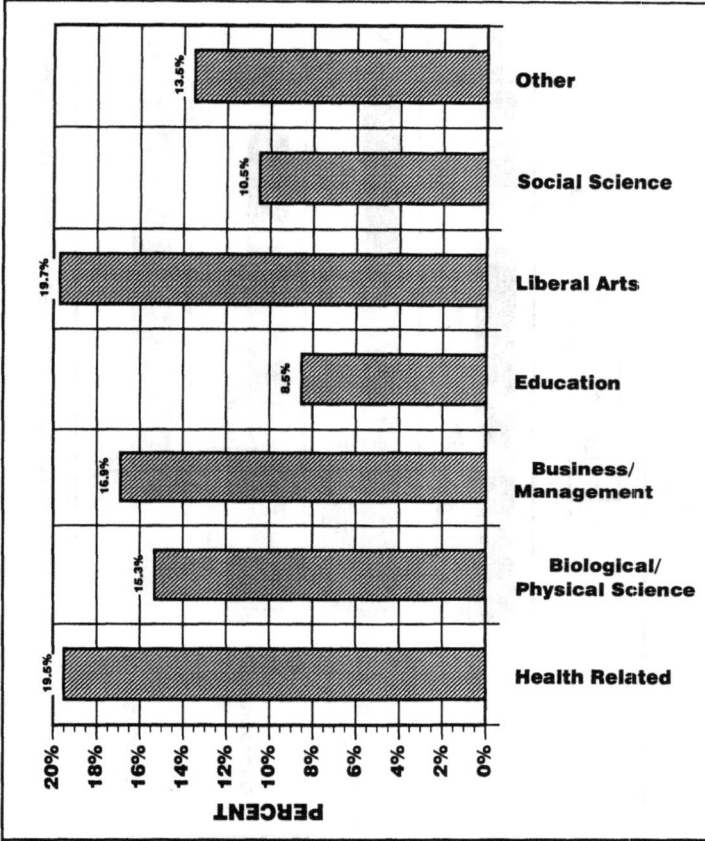

Figure 3.7   Newly Licensed Nurses' Rating of Classroom and Clinical Experiences,
              1990, 1992, 1994

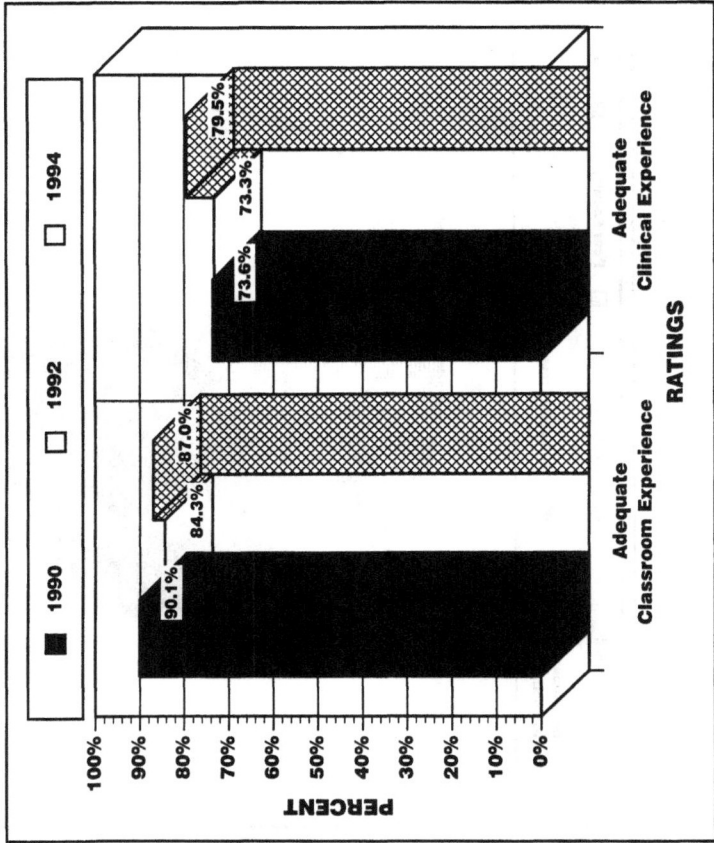

Figure 3.8   Reason for Inadequate Clinical Experience, 1994

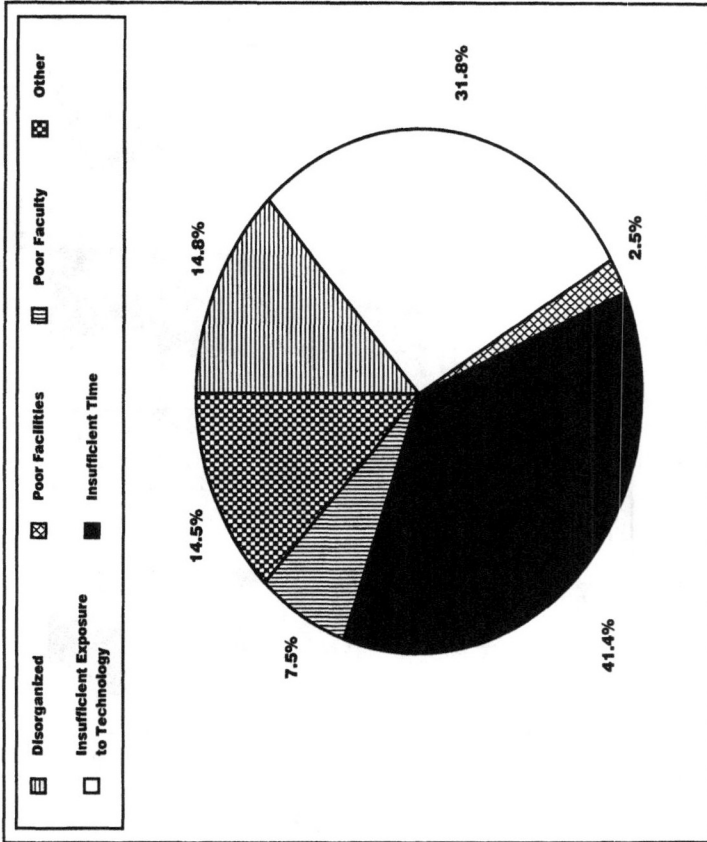

Legend:
- ▥ Disorganized
- ▨ Poor Facilities
- ▦ Poor Faculty
- ▧ Insufficient Exposure to Technology
- ◻ Insufficient Time
- ■ Other

Pie chart values: 31.8%, 2.5%, 41.4%, 7.5%, 14.5%, 14.8%

Figure 3.9   Newly Licensed Nurses Who Took the NCLEX-RN Review Course by Program Type, 1994

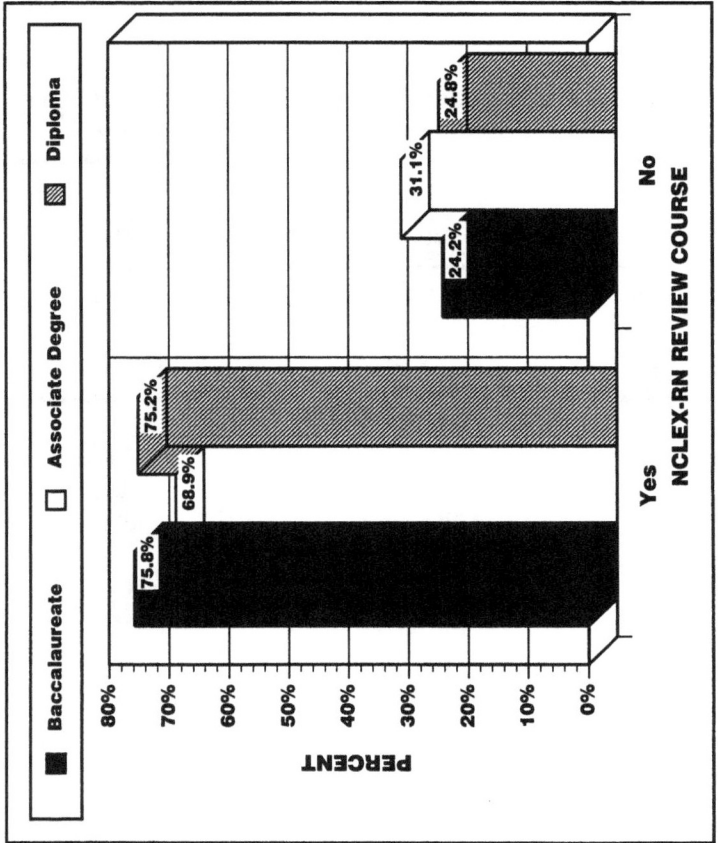

Table 3.1 Number and Percentage of Newly Licensed Nurses, by Program Type, 1990, 1992, 1994

	1990		1992		1994	
	Number	Percent	Number	Percent	Number	Percent
Diploma	2,040	8.3	2,882	8.4	3,123	7.9
Associate Degree	15,088	61.3	22,437	65.7	25,312	63.9
Baccalaureate	7,465	30.4	8,856	25.9	11,149	28.9

Table 3.2 Number of Basic RN Programs by Program Type, Region, and State, 1994

	TOTAL	PROGRAM TYPE		
		Diploma	Associate Degree	Baccalaureate
United States	**1,501**	**124**	**868**	**509**
NEW ENGLAND				
REGION TOTAL	96	11	48	37
Connecticut	17	3	6	8
Maine	15	0	8	7
Massachusetts	43	7	21	15
New Hampshire	9	0	6	3
Rhode Island	7	1	3	3
Vermont	5	0	4	1
MIDDLE ATLANTIC				
REGION TOTAL	221	51	100	70
New Jersey	37	16	14	7
New York	100	5	63	32
Pennsylvania	84	30	23	31
SOUTH ATLANTIC				
REGION TOTAL	246	18	150	78
Delaware	7	1	4	2
District of Columbia	5	0	1	4
Florida	40	1	26	13
Georgia	32	0	20	12
Maryland	24	3	14	7
North Carolina	62	4	46	12
South Carolina	20	0	13	7
Virginia	37	8	17	12
West Virginia	19	1	9	9
EAST SOUTH CENTRAL				
REGION TOTAL	129	5	78	46
Alabama	36	1	23	12
Kentucky	34	0	24	10
Mississippi	23	0	16	7
Tennessee	36	4	15	17
WEST SOUTH CENTRAL				
REGION TOTAL	150	5	86	59
Arkansas	22	2	11	9
Louisiana	23	1	9	13
Oklahoma	28	0	17	11
Texas	77	2	49	26

(continued)

Table 3.2   (continued)

	TOTAL	PROGRAM TYPE		
		Diploma	Associate Degree	Baccalaureate
EAST NORTH CENTRAL				
REGION TOTAL	267	23	148	96
Illinois	71	5	39	27
Indiana	46	1	25	20
Michigan	50	3	33	14
Ohio	69	13	34	22
Wisconsin	31	1	17	13
WEST NORTH CENTRAL				
REGION TOTAL	167	10	93	64
Iowa	40	5	23	12
Kansas	30	0	19	11
Minnesota	21	0	12	9
Missouri	46	4	27	15
Nebraska	13	1	6	6
North Dakota	7	0	0	7
South Dakota	10	0	6	4
MOUNTAIN				
REGION TOTAL	82	0	59	23
Arizona	16	0	12	4
Colorado	17	0	10	7
Idaho	7	0	5	2
Montana	5	0	3	2
Nevada	6	0	4	2
New Mexico	16	0	14	2
Utah	7	0	4	3
Wyoming	8	0	7	1
PACIFIC				
REGION TOTAL	143	1	106	36
Alaska	2	0	1	1
California	94	1	70	23
Hawaii	7	0	4	3
Oregon	16	0	13	3
Washington	24	0	18	6

Table 3.3   Number of Newly Licensed Nurses by State of Residency, Census Region, and Program Type

	TOTAL		Diploma		Associate Degree		Baccalaureate	
	Number	Percent	Number	Percent	Number	Percent	Number	Percent
GRAND TOTAL	**39,571**	**100.0**	**3,123**	**7.9**	**25,307**	**64.0**	**11,141**	**28.2**
NEW ENGLAND								
REGION TOTAL	2,294	100.0	292	12.7	1,234	53.8	768	33.5
Connecticut	498	100.0	107	21.5	204	41.0	187	37.6
Maine	251	100.0	0	0.0	157	62.5	94	37.5
Massachusetts	1,202	100.0	167	13.9	649	54.0	386	32.1
New Hampshire	39	100.0	4	10.3	19	48.7	16	41.0
Rhode Island	202	100.0	14	6.9	119	58.9	69	34.2
Vermont	102	100.0	0	0.0	86	84.3	16	15.7
MIDDLE ATLANTIC								
REGION TOTAL	6,563	100.0	1,210	18.4	3,796	57.8	1,557	23.7
New Jersey	1,174	100.0	273	23.3	603	51.4	298	25.4
New York	2,453	100.0	140	5.7	1,790	73.0	523	21.3
Pennsylvania	2,936	100.0	797	27.1	1,403	47.8	736	25.1
EAST NORTH CENTRAL								
REGION TOTAL	7,297	100.0	645	8.8	4,528	62.1	2,124	29.1
Illinois	1,787	100.0	115	6.4	1,182	66.1	490	27.4
Indiana	1,097	100.0	32	2.9	738	67.3	327	29.8

(continued)

41

Table 3.3 (continued)

	TOTAL		Diploma		PROGRAM TYPE Associate Degree		Baccalaureate	
	Number	Percent	Number	Percent	Number	Percent	Number	Percent
EAST NORTH CENTRAL *(Continued)*								
Michigan	1,363	100.0	91	6.7	895	65.7	377	27.7
Ohio	2,191	100.0	374	17.1	1,210	55.2	607	27.7
Wisconsin	859	100.0	33	3.8	503	58.6	323	37.6
WEST NORTH CENTRAL								
REGION TOTAL	3,890	100.0	333	8.6	2,268	58.3	1,289	33.1
Iowa	686	100.0	113	16.5	476	69.4	97	14.1
Kansas	581	100.0	16	2.8	342	58.9	223	38.4
Minnesota	965	100.0	0	0.0	655	67.9	310	32.1
Missouri	966	100.0	187	19.4	498	51.6	281	29.1
Nebraska	344	100.0	16	4.7	148	43.0	180	52.3
North Dakota	148	100.0	0	0.0	11	7.4	137	92.6
South Dakota	200	100.0	1	0.5	138	69.0	61	30.5
SOUTH ATLANTIC								
REGION TOTAL	6,899	100.0	369	5.3	4,736	68.6	1,794	26.0
Delaware	129	100.0	5	3.9	92	71.3	32	24.8
District of Columbia	30	100.0	0	0.0	13	43.3	17	56.7
Florida	1,565	100.0	29	1.9	1,188	75.9	348	22.2
Georgia	1,143	100.0	1	0.1	839	73.4	303	26.5

(continued)

42

Table 3.3 (continued)

	TOTAL		Diploma		PROGRAM TYPE			
					Associate Degree		Baccalaureate	
	Number	Percent	Number	Percent	Number	Percent	Number	Percent
SOUTH ATLANTIC *(continued)*								
Maryland	741	100.0	56	7.6	438	59.1	247	33.3
North Carolina	1,320	100.0	96	7.3	885	67.0	339	25.7
South Carolina	535	100.0	4	0.7	382	71.4	149	27.9
Virginia	1,009	100.0	149	14.8	583	57.8	277	27.5
West Virginia	427	100.0	29	6.8	316	74.0	82	19.2
EAST SOUTH CENTRAL								
REGION TOTAL	3,245	100.0	105	3.2	2,323	71.6	817	25.2
Alabama	757	100.0	23	3.0	542	71.6	192	25.4
Kentucky	926	100.0	2	0.2	695	75.1	229	24.7
Mississippi	554	100.0	5	0.9	421	76.0	128	23.1
Tennessee	1,008	100.0	75	7.4	665	66.0	268	26.6
WEST SOUTH CENTRAL								
REGION TOTAL	4,137	100.0	107	2.6	2,772	67.0	1,258	30.4
Arkansas	454	100.0	8	1.8	335	73.8	111	24.4
Louisiana	644	100.0	0	0.0	327	50.8	317	49.2
Oklahoma	616	100.0	0	0.0	403	65.4	213	34.6
Texas	2,423	100.0	99	4.1	1,707	70.4	617	25.5

(continued)

43

Table 3.3 (continued)

	TOTAL		Diploma		PROGRAM TYPE Associate Degree		Baccalaureate	
	Number	Percent	Number	Percent	Number	Percent	Number	Percent
MOUNTAIN								
REGION TOTAL	1,954	100.0	2	0.1	1,358	69.5	594	30.2
Arizona	380	100.0	2	0.5	280	73.7	98	25.8
Colorado	486	100.0	0	0.0	262	53.9	224	46.1
Idaho	184	100.0	0	0.0	140	76.1	44	23.9
Montana	124	100.0	0	0.0	68	54.8	56	45.2
Nevada	112	100.0	0	0.0	66	58.9	46	41.1
New Mexico	189	100.0	0	0.0	159	84.1	30	21.3
Utah	317	100.0	0	0.0	252	79.5	65	20.5
Wyoming	162	100.0	0	0.0	131	80.9	31	19.1
PACIFIC								
REGION TOTAL	3,292	100.0	60	1.8	2,292	69.6	940	28.6
Alaska	35	100.0	0	0.0	17	48.6	18	51.4
California	2,125	100.0	59	2.8	1,482	69.7	584	27.5
Hawaii	9	100.0	0	0.0	2	22.2	7	77.8
Oregon	489	100.0	0	0.0	330	67.5	159	32.5
Washington	634	100.0	1	.2	461	72.7	172	27.1

Table 3.4 Highest Earned Credential of Newly Licensed Nurses Who Held College Degrees Prior to Nursing School, by Program Type, 1994

| | TOTAL | | HIGHEST EARNED COLLEGE CREDENTIAL | | | | | | | |
| | | | Associate Degree | | Bachelor's Degree | | Master's Degree | | Doctoral Degree | |
	Number	Percent	Number	Percent	Number	Percent	Number	Percent	Number	Percent
TOTAL	8,071	100.0	3,471	43.0	4,143	51.3	417	5.2	40	.5
PROGRAM TYPE										
Diploma	605	100.0	227	37.5	355	58.7	23	3.8	0	.0
Associate Degree	4,779	100.0	2,397	50.2	2,124	44.4	239	5.0	19	.4
Baccalaureate	2,687	100.0	847	31.5	1,664	61.9	155	5.8	21	.8

Table 3.5   Adequacy of Nursing Education by Program Type, 1994

	Adequate		Not Adequate	
	Number	Percent	Number	Percent
CLASSROOM EXPERIENCE				
Diploma	2,626	92.5	210	7.4
Associate Degree	18,742	83.8	3,636	16.2
Baccalaureate	8,482	84.6	1,545	15.4
CLINICAL EXPERIENCE				
Diploma	2,532	91.0	248	8.9
Associate Degree	15,941	72.8	5,948	27.2
Baccalaureate	7,402	74.2	2,507	25.3

Table 3.6 Reason for Fair or Poor Rating of Clinical Experiences by Newly Licensed Nurses, by Program Type, 1994

	PROGRAM TYPE					
	Diploma		Associate Degree		Baccalaureate	
	Number	Percent	Number	Percent	Number	Percent
Reason for Poor Rating						
Disorganized-Fragmented Use of Time	27	11.3	838	14.4	389	15.9
Insufficient Time	86	36.0	2,401	41.4	1,024	41.8
Insufficient Exposure to Technology	75	31.4	1,895	32.7	728	29.7
Poor Faculty	19	7.9	451	7.8	165	6.7
Poor Facilities	4	1.7	149	2.6	56	2.3
Other	56	23.4	816	14.1	356	14.5

4

EMPLOYMENT DISTRIBUTION

The increased responsibility of patient care was daunting, but administration has demanded a patient load of 6 to 7 patients per nurse without any help from aides, etc. I feel overwhelmed and inadequate most of the time. I also fear I will lose my licensure due to inadequate and compromised care. Is this the future of nursing? (Oregon)

I think graduates from nursing school today will have to be more flexible in their options for work and be willing to move to find experience and employment.   *(Ohio)*

Respondents commented most frequently about employment issues, and some even wrote letters and attached them to their surveys. They reported on their employment status, job searches, employment settings, positions held, activity levels, and salaries.

EMPLOYMENT STATUS

Although only 1.2 percent of newly licensed nurses were not employed in nursing in 1994 (Figure 4.1), this figure represents an increase from 1992 when 0.3 of the respondents were not employed in nursing. The increase in unemployment occurred among all types of programs, with the greatest increase among associate degree graduates.

The most common reason newly licensed nurses were not employed in nursing was a lack of jobs available to them (Figure 4.2). Other reasons included not being able to find the jobs they wanted, continuing education, and family responsibilities. More diploma nurses reported that they could not find what they wanted than graduates of other program types (Table 4.3), and none of the diploma nurses cited continuing education as a reason for not being employed in nursing.

Of all newly licensed nurses who were employed in nursing, most reported that they were not seeking other employment (Table 4.2). There was an increase in the number of those who were seeking other employment in 1994 (27.6%) compared with those in 1992 (23.7 %). The percentage of nurses seeking other nursing jobs was 27.6 percent while 1.0 percent were seeking non-nursing jobs. By program type, diploma nurses were more likely to be seeking other nursing jobs, and baccalaureate nurses were more likely to be seeking non-nursing jobs.

FINDING JOBS

The length of time it took for respondents to find their first jobs was longer than in previous years (Figure 4.3). Although most graduates continued to find jobs before graduation, the proportion of those who did so decreased dramatically. More baccalaureate graduates found jobs before graduation than associate degree or diploma graduates. Of the baccalaureate graduates, 78.5 percent found jobs one month after graduation, compared with 77.4 percent of the associate degree and 75.7 percent of the diploma graduates (Table 4.4).

Nurses in the West South Central region found jobs before graduation at a higher rate than nurses in other regions (Figure 4.4). Nurses in the Pacific region found fewer jobs before graduation and were not able to find jobs as quickly as nurses in other regions.

Respondents reported very few jobs available to them after graduation (Figure 4.5). There has been a consistent pattern in the decline of jobs since 1990.

Nurses' perceptions of job availability were similar among program types (Figure 4.6). Of the nurses who perceived that many jobs were available, most were associate degree graduates. Few diploma graduates reported that many jobs were available.

Fewer baccalaureate graduates took jobs at clinical sites than associate degree or diploma graduates (Figure 4.7). Most baccalaureate and associate degree nurses found jobs through prior association with an institution. Other methods of finding jobs included classified ads, word-of-mouth, faculty recommendations, and on-site recruitment.

A large proportion of graduates of all program types found jobs through word-of-mouth. Very few nurses within any program type found jobs through employment agencies.

EMPLOYMENT SETTINGS

Most new graduates found employment in hospitals, although there has been an increase in the number of new graduates finding jobs in settings other than hospitals since 1990 (Figure 4.8). Of those working in hospitals, most graduates from all three programs took positions in medical-surgical units of hospitals (Figure 4.10). Very few worked in emergency rooms or on obstetric/gynecological or pediatric units, and the smallest percentage of nurses worked in operating rooms. More diploma nurses (43%) worked in emergency rooms than baccalaureate (3.6%) or associate degree (6.0%) nurses (Figure 4.10).

Only 18.9 percent of all newly licensed nurses were employed in settings other than hospitals (Table 4.6). A greater proportion of associate degree graduates (22.8%) found employment outside hospital settings than baccalaureate (11.6%) or diploma (14.3%) graduates. Of those respondents (11.4%) who were employed by nursing homes, 80.3% were associate degree program graduates. Of the 4.8 percent employed in community, home, or public health agencies, 67.6 percent were also associate degree nurses.

Positions Held

Most respondents held general duty/staff positions in all employment settings, particularly in hospitals (Figure 4.9). Newly licensed nurses were more likely to be head or assistant head nurses in nursing home settings.

Respondents were asked why they chose their current positions. Almost half (44.0%) chose their current positions because of their choice of specialty, and this was the most common reason reported across all program types (Table 4.5). Thirty eight percent chose their current jobs because of salary/benefits. The least reported reason was for housing near the employment site.

Activity Level

A preponderance of newly licensed nurses were working full-time (81.2%), but this number is down from two years ago (Figure 4.11). Few respondents worked less than 20 hours per week or per diem (Figure 4.12). By employment setting, a larger percentage of per diem nurses worked in community/home/public health agencies while the largest percentage of part-time nurses worked in schools or physicians' offices (Figure 4.13).

Although the vast majority of newly licensed nurses continue to work full-time, the number is on the decline in all employment settings (Table 4.7). In 1992, 85.8 percent of newly licensed nurses worked full-time, compared with 1994 when 81.2 percent reported full-time employment. Associate degree nurses who were married with children were more likely to work per diem than their counterparts from other programs (Table 4.8).

SALARIES

Figures 4.14 through 4.16 illustrate the salaries of new nurses by region, state, and employment. Overall, salaries have increased in the past two years. The mean salary for all regions in 1994 was $29,384, an increase of $798 from 1992. The highest mean salary for full-time nurses was in the Middle Atlantic region at $33,182 and the lowest was in the West North Central at $26,032. Slight decreases in mean average full-time salaries were found only in New England and the Pacific regions.

Generally, diploma nurses earned the highest salaries, earning an average of $30,189 for full-time employment (Table 4.9). In general, mean full-time salaries increased for all regions, states, and program types. New Jersey nurses earned the highest full-time salaries, followed by Connecticut.

The mean part-time salary for all regions was $20,756 (Figure 4.15) but varied from state to state and region to region. The region with the highest mean part-time salary was the Pacific region ($23,894), and the lowest was in the West North Central ($18,816). The state with the highest mean part-time salary was California ($26,484), and the lowest was Arkansas ($18,391). Generally, nurses in states with major cities or located near metropolitan areas earned higher salaries than states with large rural communities.

Per diem salaries were comparable to those of full-time and part-time employed nurses. The mean salary for all per diem nurses was $24,283 (Figure 4.16). The region with the highest salary for this group was the Pacific ($26,485), and the lowest was the West North Central ($18,763).

Figure 4.1   Employment Status of Newly Licensed Nurses, 1990, 1992, 1994

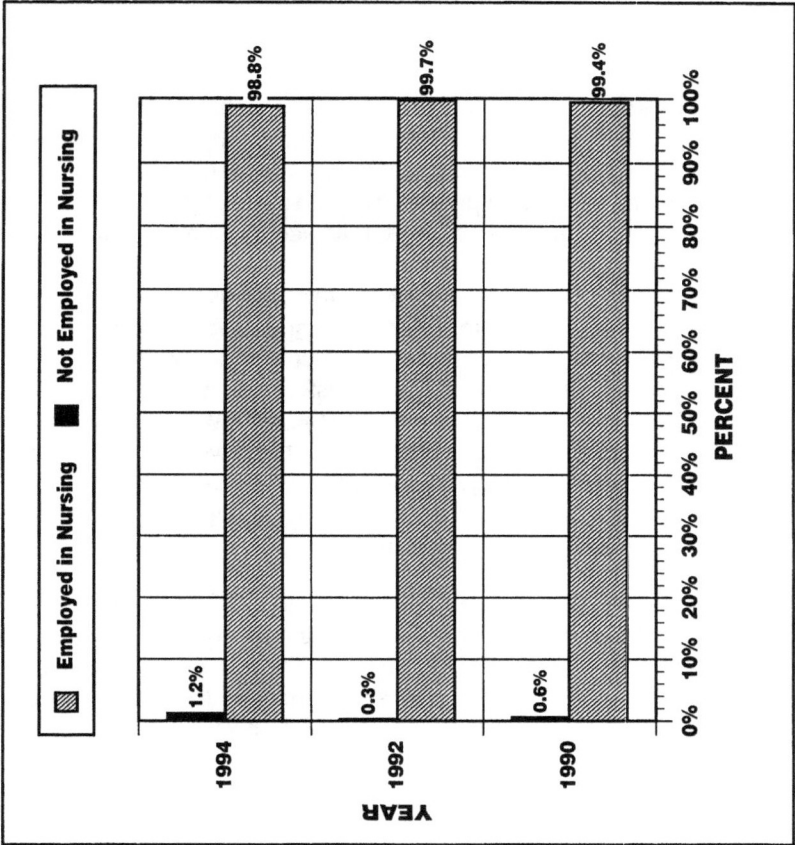

Figure 4.2   Reason Why Newly Licensed Nurses Were Not Employed in Nursing by Program Type, 1994

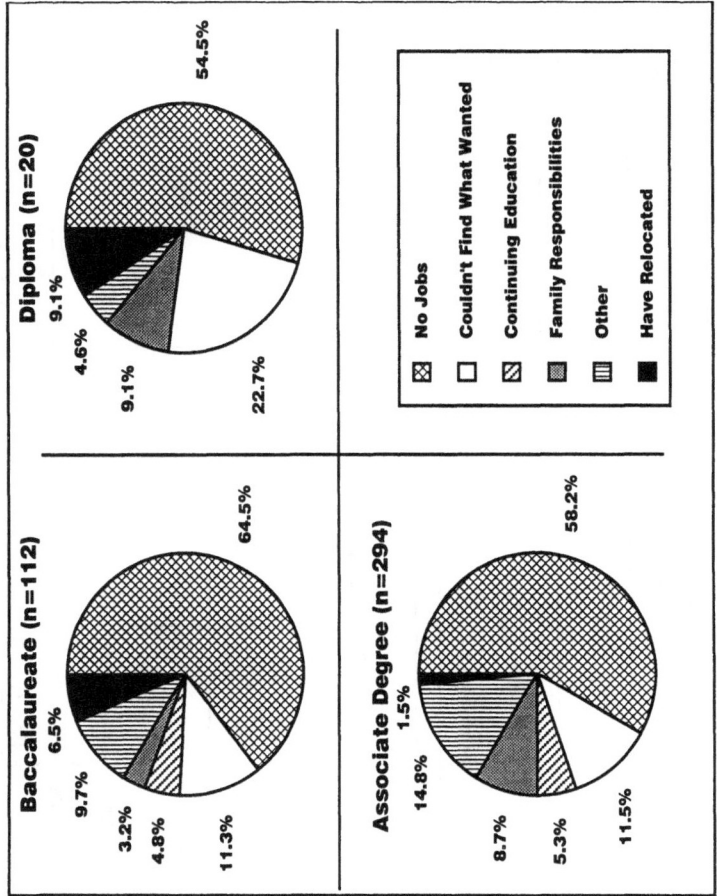

55

Figure 4.3 Length of Time for Newly Licensed Nurses to Find First Job, 1982, 1988, 1990, 1992, 1994

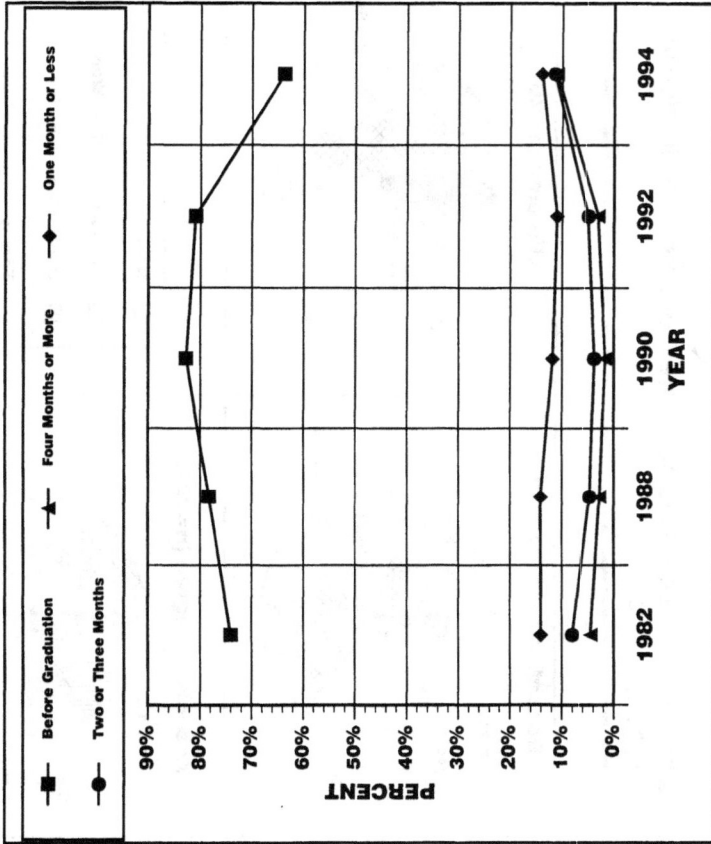

Figure 4.4 Length of Time to Find First Job by Census Region, 1994

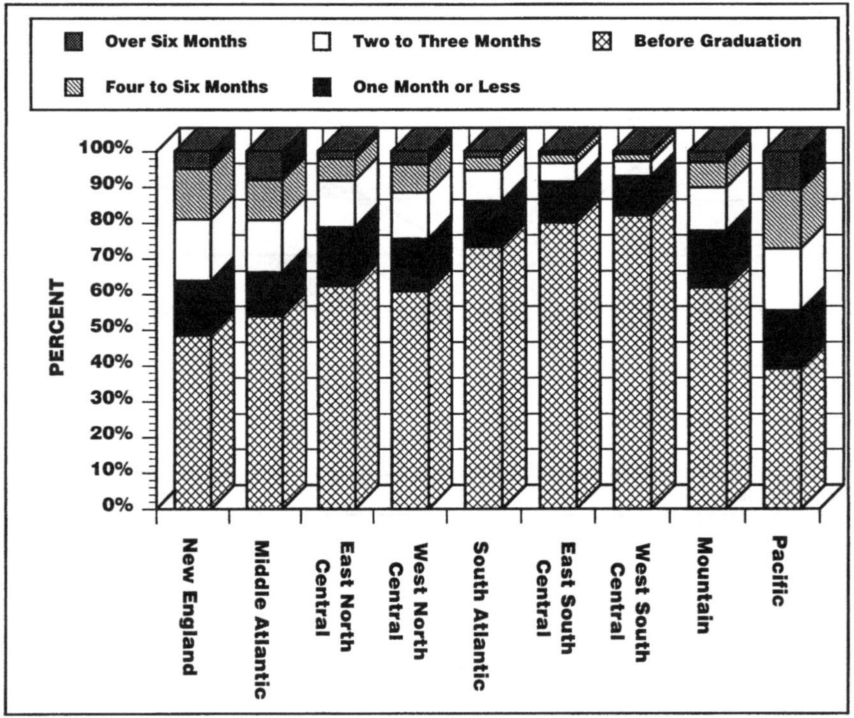

Over Six Months
Two to Three Months
Before Graduation
Four to Six Months
One Month or Less
PERCENT
100%
90%
80%
70%
60%
50%
40%
30%
20%
10%
0%
New England
Middle Atlantic
East North Central
West North Central
South Atlantic
East South Central
West South Central
Mountain
Pacific

Figure 4.5 Perception of Job Availability, 1990, 1992, 1994

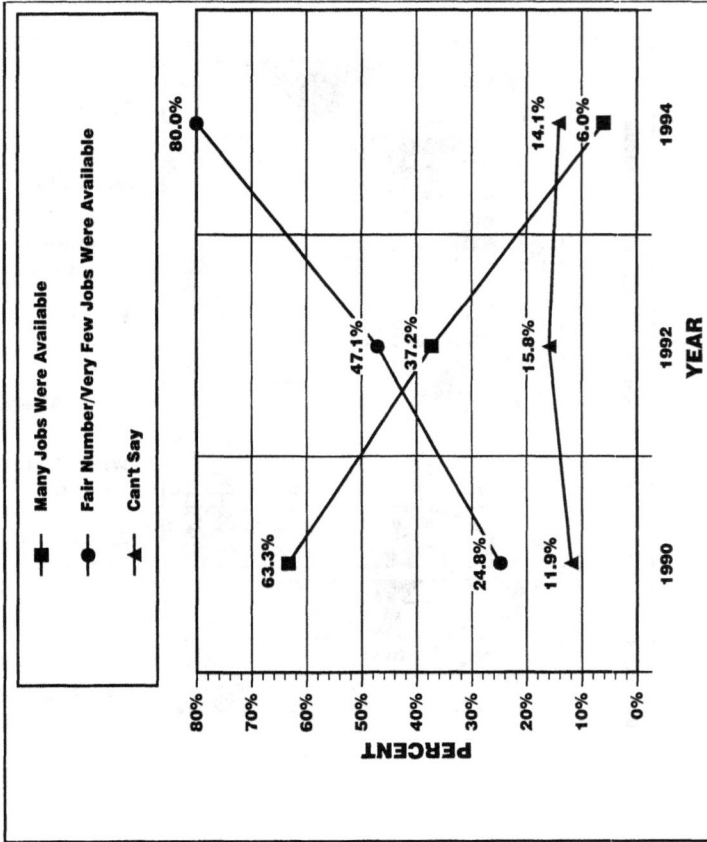

Legend:
- ■ Many Jobs Were Available
- ● Fair Number/Very Few Jobs Were Available
- ▲ Can't Say

Data points:
- Many Jobs Were Available: 63.3% (1990), 37.2% (1992), 6.0% (1994)
- Fair Number/Very Few Jobs Were Available: 24.8% (1990), 47.1% (1992), 80.0% (1994)
- Can't Say: 11.9% (1990), 15.8% (1992), 14.1% (1994)

Y-axis: PERCENT (0% to 80%)
X-axis: YEAR (1990, 1992, 1994)

Figure 4.6 Newly Licensed Nurses' Perception of Job Availability by Program Type, 1994

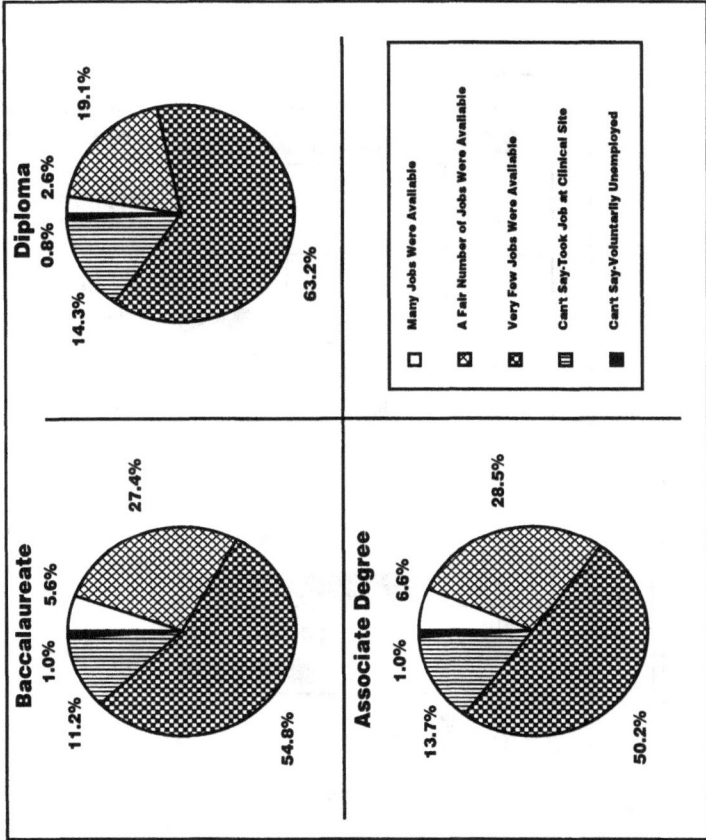

Baccalaureate
1.0%
5.6%
27.4%
11.2%
54.8%

Diploma
0.8% 2.6%
19.1%
14.3%
63.2%

Associate Degree
1.0%
6.6%
28.5%
13.7%
50.2%

☐ Many Jobs Were Available
☒ A Fair Number of Jobs Were Available
☒ Very Few Jobs Were Available
▥ Can't Say-Took Job at Clinical Site
■ Can't Say-Voluntarily Unemployed

Figure 4.7 How Newly Licensed Nurses Found Their Current Jobs by Program Type, 1994

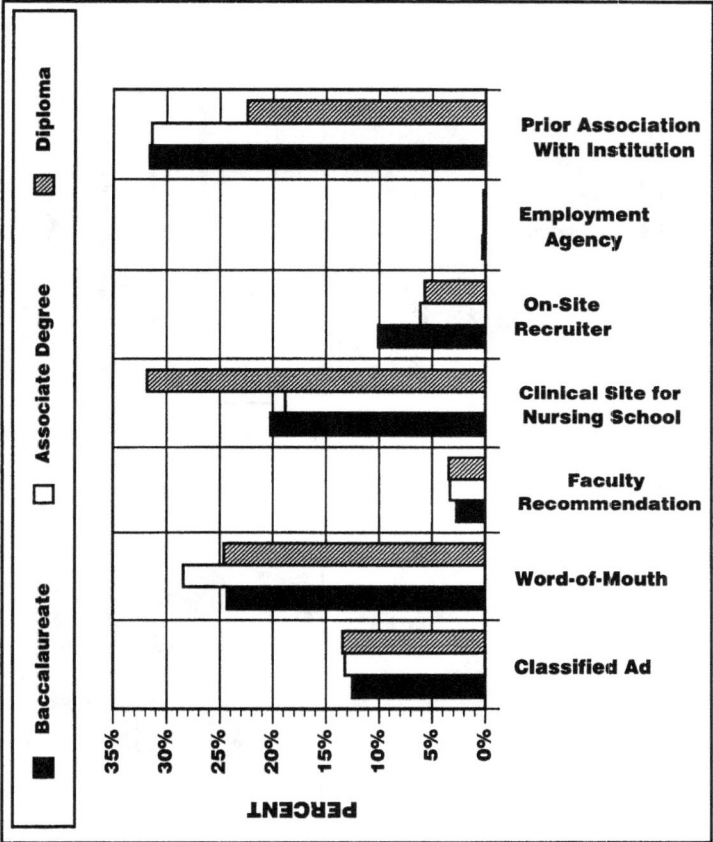

Figure 4.8 Employment Settings of Newly Licensed Nurses, 1982, 1988, 1990, 1992, 1994

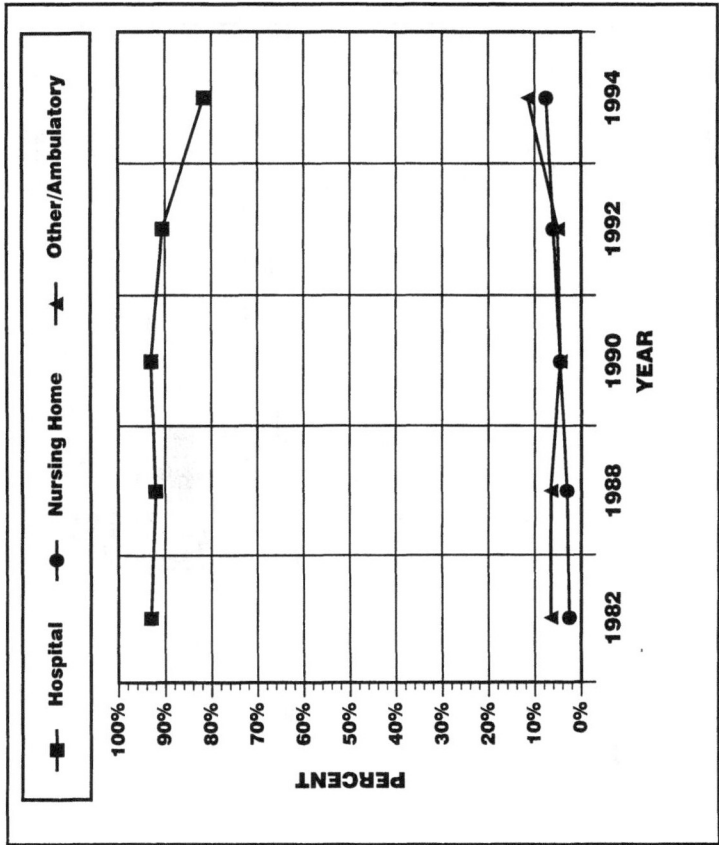

61

Figure 4.9   Type of Position by Employment Setting, 1994

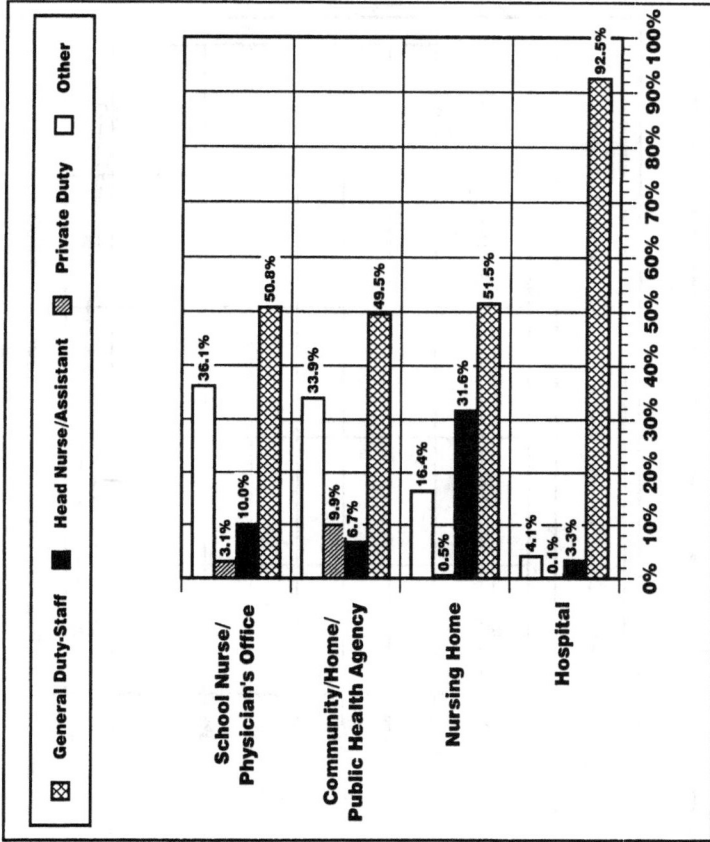

Legend: General Duty-Staff · Head Nurse/Assistant · Private Duty · Other

School Nurse/Physician's Office: 3.1%, 10.0%, 36.1%, 50.8%

Community/Home/Public Health Agency: 9.9%, 6.7%, 33.9%, 49.5%

Nursing Home: 0.5%, 31.6%, 16.4%, 51.5%

Hospital: 4.1%, 0.1%, 3.3%, 92.5%

Figure 4.10 Hospital Units Where Newly Licensed Nurses Worked by Program Type, 1994

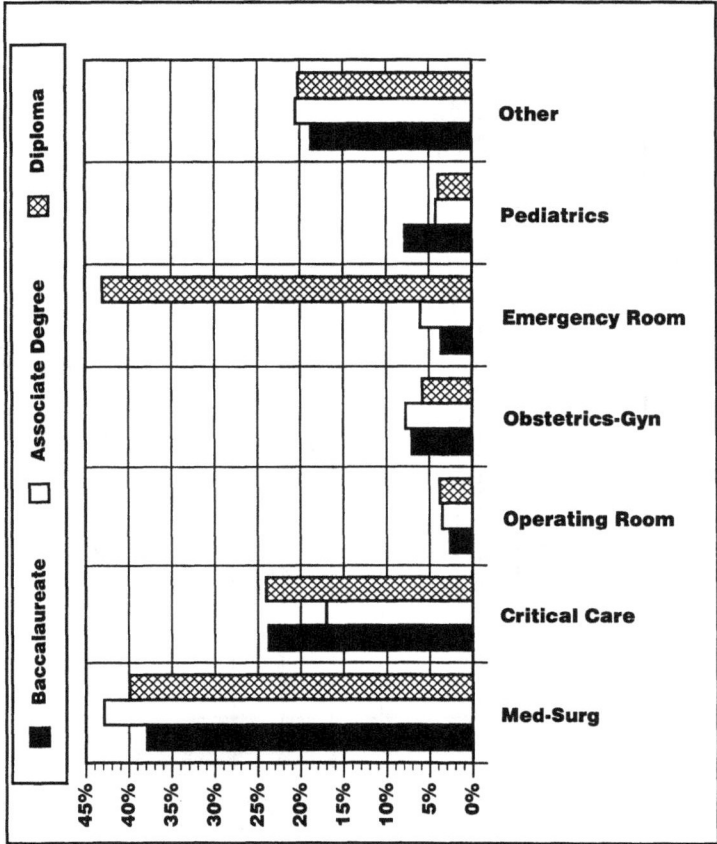

Figure 4.11 Newly Licensed Nurses' Activity Status, 1990, 1992, 1994

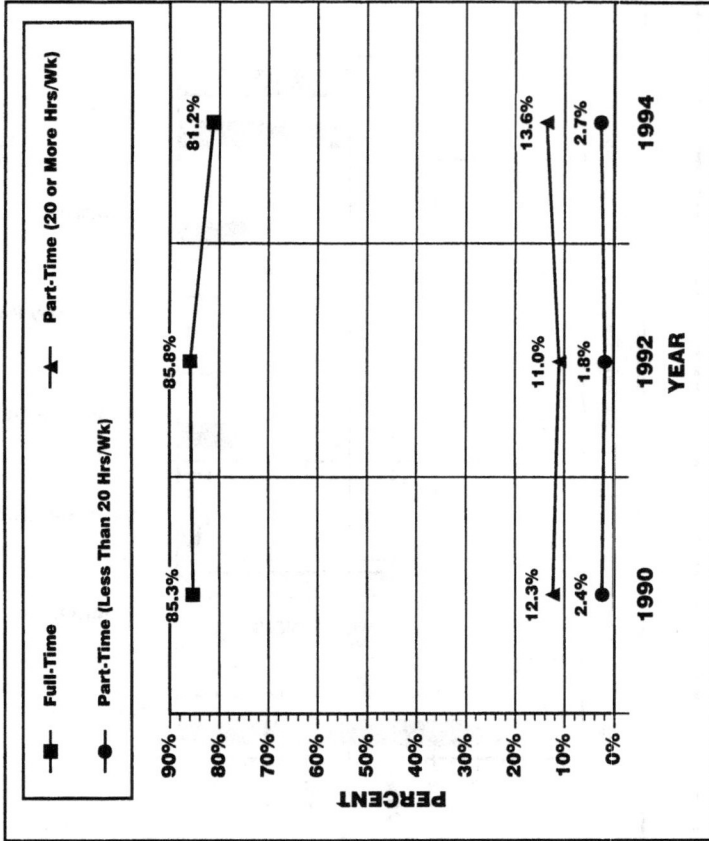

64

Figure 4.12 Newly Licensed Nurses' Activity Status by Program Type, 1994

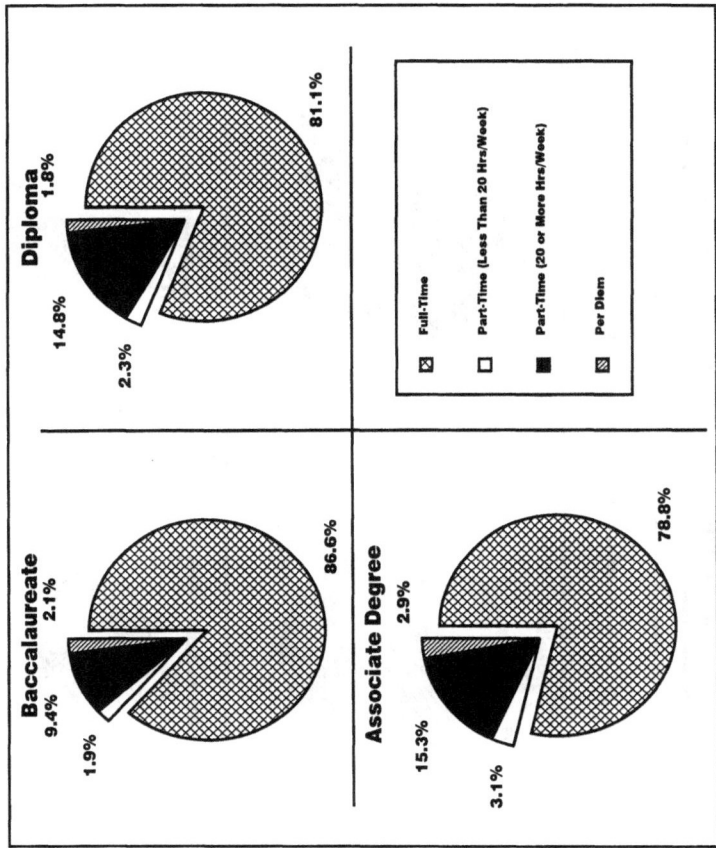

Baccalaureate

9.4%
1.9%
2.1%
86.6%

Diploma

14.8%
2.3%
1.8%
81.1%

Associate Degree

15.3%
3.1%
2.9%
78.8%

Legend:
☒ Full-Time
☐ Part-Time (Less Than 20 Hrs/Week)
■ Part-Time (20 or More Hrs/Week)
▨ Per Diem

Figure 4.13 Newly Licensed Nurses' Activity by Employment Setting, 1994

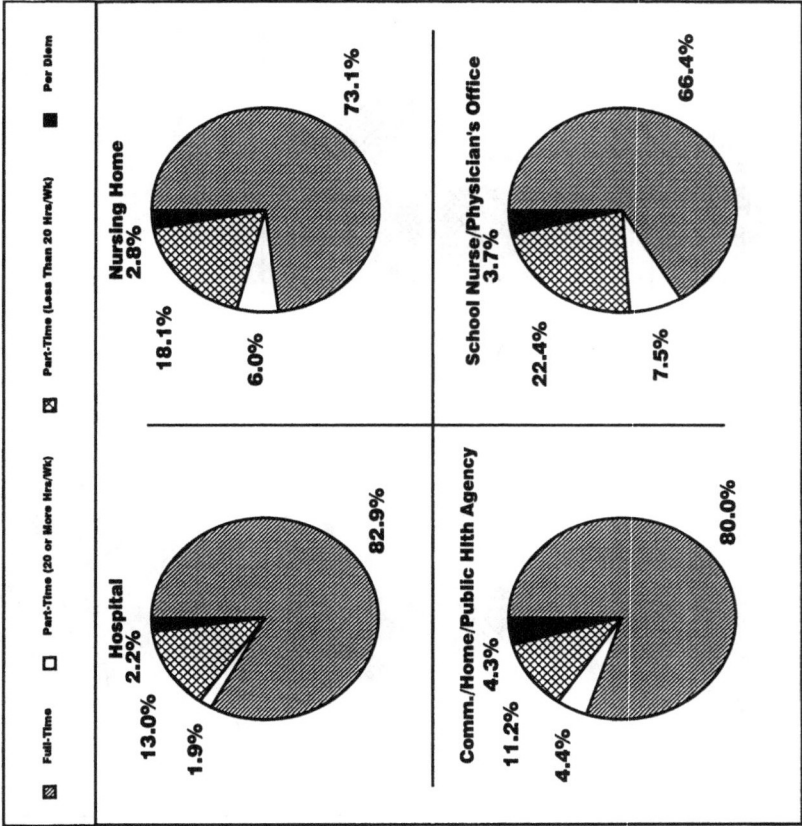

Legend: Full-Time ▨   Part-Time (20 or More Hrs/Wk) ☐   Part-Time (Less Than 20 Hrs/Wk) ▧   Per Diem ■

Hospital
2.2%
13.0%
1.9%
82.9%

Nursing Home
2.8%
18.1%
6.0%
73.1%

Comm./Home/Public Hlth Agency
4.3%
11.2%
4.4%
80.0%

School Nurse/Physician's Office
3.7%
22.4%
7.5%
66.4%

Figure 4.14 Mean Full-Time Salaries of Newly Licensed Nurses by Region

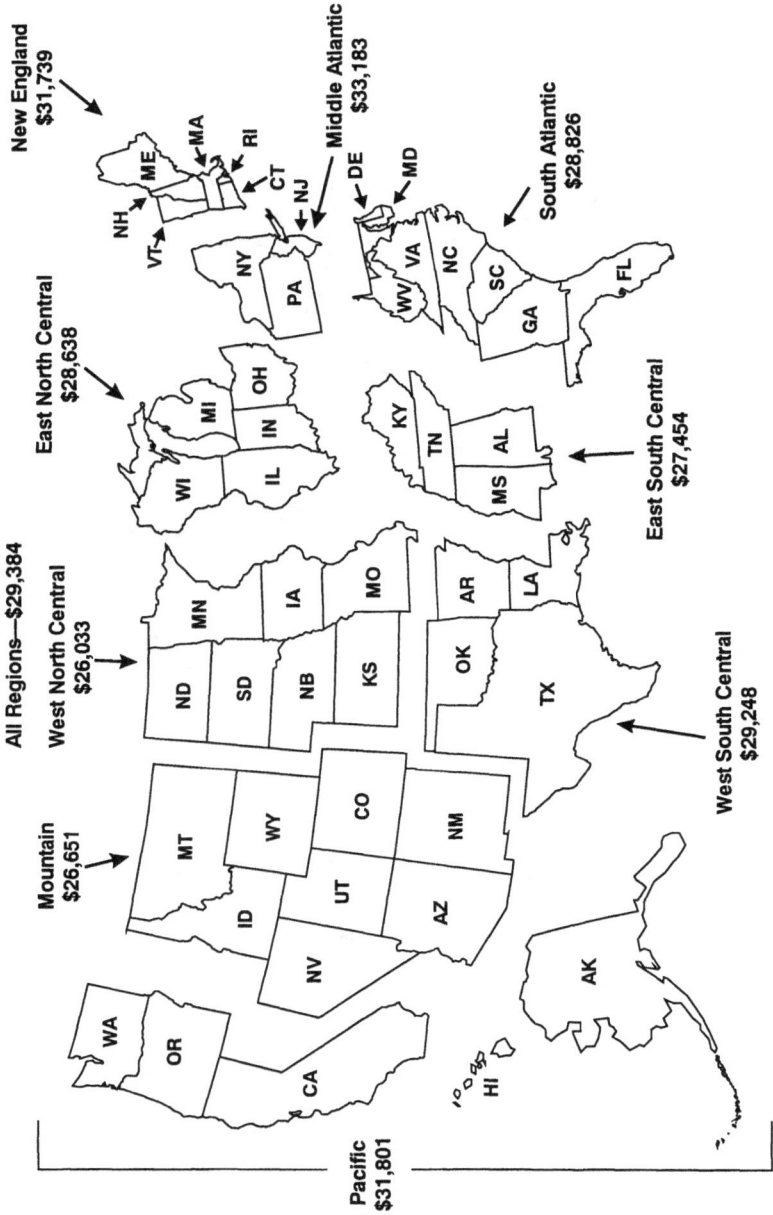

All Regions—$29,384

New England $31,739

Middle Atlantic $33,183

South Atlantic $28,826

East North Central $28,638

East South Central $27,454

West North Central $26,033

West South Central $29,248

Mountain $26,651

Pacific $31,801

67

Figure 4.15 Mean Part-Time Salaries of Newly Licensed Nurses by Region

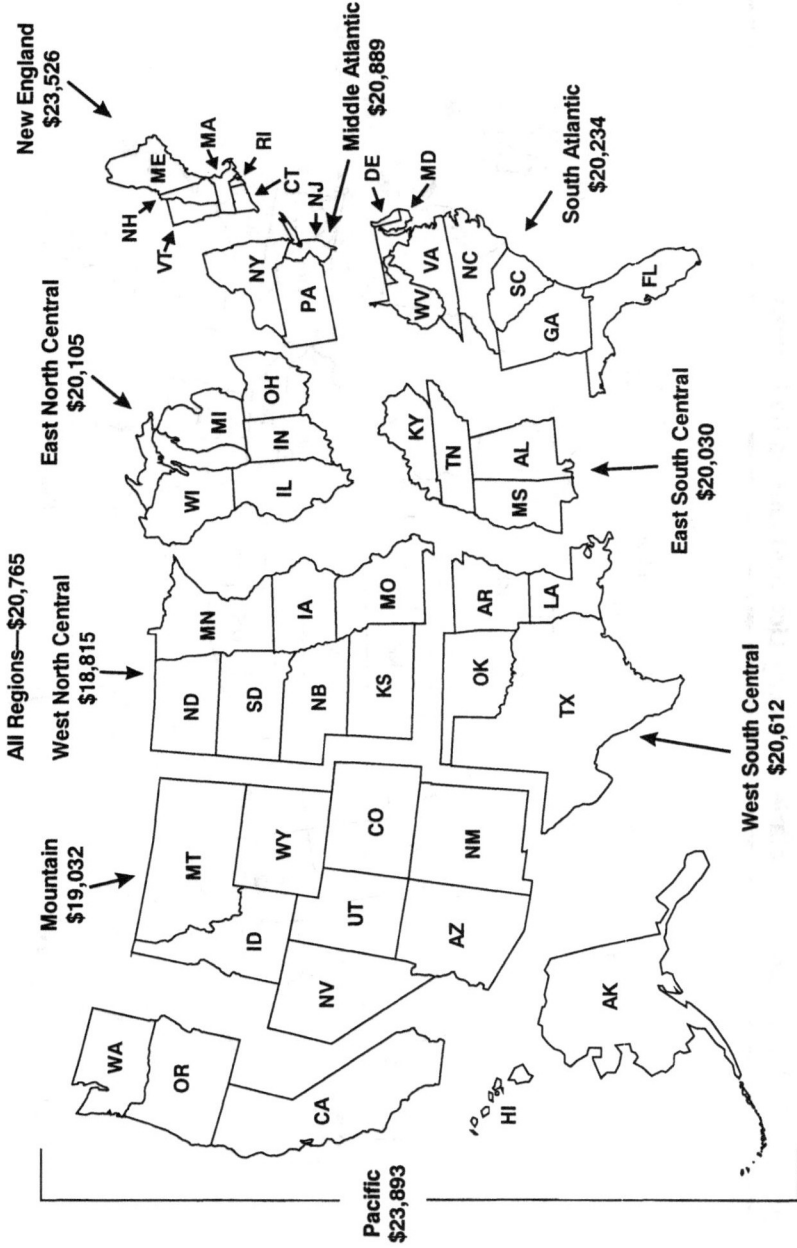

New England
$23,526

Middle Atlantic
$20,889

South Atlantic
$20,234

East North Central
$20,105

East South Central
$20,030

All Regions—$20,765

West North Central
$18,815

West South Central
$20,612

Mountain
$19,032

Pacific
$23,893

MA
RI
CT
NJ
ME
NH
VT
NY
PA
DE
MD
WV
VA
NC
SC
GA
FL

WI
MI
IL
IN
OH

KY
TN
AL
MS

ND
SD
NB
KS
MN
IA
MO
OK
AR
TX
LA

MT
ID
WY
UT
CO
NV
AZ
NM

WA
OR
CA
AK
HI

Figure 4.16 Mean Per-Diem Salaries of Newly Licensed Nurses by Region

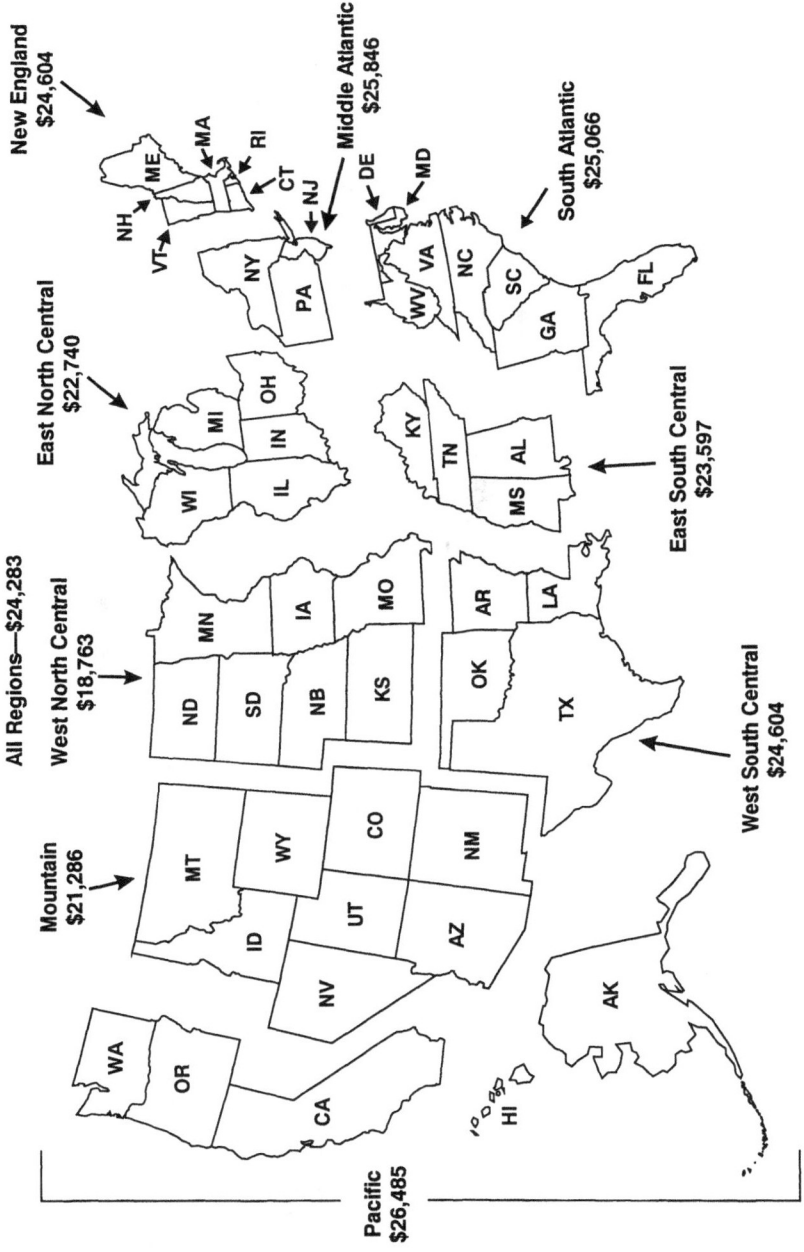

New England
$24,604

Middle Atlantic
$25,846

South Atlantic
$25,066

East North Central
$22,740

East South Central
$23,597

All Regions—$24,283

West North Central
$18,763

Mountain
$21,286

West South Central
$24,604

Pacific
$26,485

Table 4.1 Employment Status of Newly Licensed Nurses by Program Type, 1990, 1992, 1994

| | EMPLOYMENT STATUS | | | | | |
| | Percent Employed in Nursing | | | Percent Not Employed in Nursing | | |
	1990	1992	1994	1990	1992	1994
TOTAL	99.4	99.7	98.8	0.6	0.3	1.2
PROGRAM TYPE						
Diploma	99.8	99.7	99.3	0.2	0.3	0.7
Associate Degree	99.4	99.7	98.7	0.6	0.3	1.3
Baccalaureate	99.4	99.7	98.9	0.6	0.3	1.1

Table 4.2   Newly Licensed Nurses Employed in Nursing—Employment Status
by Program Type, 1994

EMPLOYMENT STATUS

PROGRAM TYPE	TOTAL		Not Seeking Other Job		Seeking Other Nursing Job		Seeking A Non-Nursing Job	
	Number	Percent	Number	Percent	Number	Percent	Number	Percent
TOTAL	35,554	100.0	25,393	71.4	9,802	27.6	359	1.0
Diploma	2,855	100.0	2,005	70.2	828	29.0	22	0.8
Associate Degree	22,597	100.0	16,183	71.6	6,199	27.4	215	1.0
Baccalaureate	10,102	100.0	7,205	71.3	2,775	27.5	122	1.2

Table 4.3 Main Reason Why Newly Licensed Nurses Were Not Employed in Nursing, by Program Type, 1994

	PROGRAM TYPE					
	Diploma		Associate Degree		Baccalaureate	
	Number	Percent	Number	Percent	Number	Percent
TOTAL	20	100.0	294	100.0	112	100.0
REASON						
No Jobs	12	60.0	188	63.9	80	71.4
Jobs Not What Wanted	5	25.0	37	12.6	14	12.5
Continuing Education	0	0.0	17	5.8	6	5.4
Family Responsibilities	2	10.0	28	9.5	4	3.6
Other	1	5.0	48	16.3	12	10.7
Have Relocated	2	10.0	5	1.7	8	7.1
Don't Want to Practice	0	0.0	1	0.3	0	0.0

Table 4.4 Length of Time to Find First Nursing Job by Program Type, 1990, 1992, 1994

	1990	1992	1994
Found Job Before Graduation			
TOTAL	**82.7**	**80.9**	**63.7**
Diploma	89.6	87.5	64.4
Associate Degree	81.3	79.5	62.7
Baccalaureate	83.6	82.3	65.6
Found Job 1 Month or Less			
TOTAL	**11.8**	**11.0**	**13.9**
Diploma	6.5	7.6	11.3
Associate Degree	13.0	11.9	14.7
Baccalaureate	10.9	9.6	12.9
Found Job 2-3 Months			
TOTAL	**3.8**	**5.0**	**11.4**
Diploma	2.8	3.4	12.3
Associate Degree	3.9	5.2	11.6
Baccalaureate	4.0	5.0	10.9
Found Job 4 or More Months			
TOTAL	**1.7**	**3.1**	**11.0**
Diploma	1.1	1.6	12.0
Associate Degree	1.8	3.4	11.1
Baccalaureate	1.6	3.0	10.6

Table 4.5 Reasons for Choosing Current Position by Type of Nursing Education of Newly Licensed Nurses, 1994

	PROGRAM TYPE							
	TOTAL		Diploma		Associate Degree		Baccalaureate	
	Number	Percent	Number	Percent	Number	Percent	Number	Percent
TOTAL	34,701	100.0	2,781	100.0	22,027	100.0	9,893	100.0
REASONS FOR CHOOSING POSITION								
Vacation	1,839	5.3	134	4.8	1,220	5.5	485	4.9
Housing	505	1.5	31	1.1	304	1.4	170	1.7
Health Insurance	3,779	10.9	313	11.3	2,593	11.8	873	8.8
Tuition Reimbursement	3,596	10.4	410	14.7	2,121	9.6	1,065	10.8
Salary-Benefits	13,376	38.5	1,028	37.0	8,840	40.1	3,508	35.5
Promotional Opportunities	2,572	7.4	170	6.1	1,649	7.5	753	7.6
Had Externship There	4,336	12.5	334	12.0	2,281	10.4	1,721	17.4
Desired This Specialization	15,252	44.0	1,273	45.8	9,264	42.1	4,715	47.7
Other	12,517	36.1	978	35.2	7,975	36.2	3,564	36.0

Table 4.6 Employment Setting of Newly Licensed Nurses by Program Type, 1994

SETTING	TOTAL		Diploma		Associate Degree		Baccalaureate	
	Number	Percent	Number	Percent	Number	Percent	Number	Percent
TOTAL	33,577	100.0	2,732	100.0	21,238	100.0	9,607	100.0
Hospital	27,440	81.7	2,353	86.1	16,556	78.0	8,531	88.8
Nursing Home	3,813	11.4	254	9.3	3,060	14.4	499	5.2
Community/Home or Public Health Agency	1,610	4.8	81	3.0	1,088	5.1	441	4.6
School Nurse/ Physician's Office	923	2.7	54	2.0	698	3.3	171	1.8

Table 4.7 Activity Status of Newly Licensed Nurses by Employment Setting, 1994

			ACTIVITY STATUS							
	TOTAL		Full-Time		Part-Time—Less Than 20 Hours/Week		Part-Time—20 Or More Hours/Week		Work As Needed /Per Diem	
	Number	Percent	Number	Percent	Number	Percent	Number	Percent	Number	Percent
TOTAL	**33,529**	**100.0**	**27,239**	**81.2**	**874**	**2.6**	**4,604**	**13.7**	**812**	**2.4**
EMPLOYMENT SETTING										
Hospital	27,270	100.0	22,616	82.9	509	1.9	3,542	13.0	603	2.2
Nursing Home	3,759	100.0	2,746	73.1	227	6.0	680	18.1	106	2.8
Community, Home or Public Health Agency	1,593	100.0	1,275	80.0	70	4.4	179	11.2	69	4.3
School Nurse or Physician's Office	907	100.0	602	66.4	68	7.5	203	22.4	34	3.7

Table 4.8 Activity Status of Newly Licensed Nurses by Marital Status, Presence of Children, and Program Type, 1994

| | TOTAL | | ACTIVITY STATUS | | | | | |
| | | | Full-Time | | Part-Time | | Per Diem | |
	Number	Percent	Number	Percent	Number	Percent	Number	Percent
MARITAL STATUS								
Married W. Child	12,300	100.0	8,959	72.8	2,455	24.0	390	3.2
Married No Child	6,059	100.0	5,121	84.5	799	13.1	139	2.3
Not Married W. Child	3,808	100.0	3,215	84.4	495	13.0	98	2.6
Not Married No Child	9,258	100.0	8,144	88.0	929	10.0	185	2.0
PROGRAM TYPE								
DIPLOMA								
Married W. Child	833	100.0	602	72.3	218	26.2	13	1.6
Married No Child	453	100.0	377	83.2	68	15.0	8	1.8
Not Married W. Child	290	100.0	247	85.2	36	12.4	7	2.4
Not Married No Child	922	100.0	795	86.2	110	11.9	17	1.8
ASSOCIATE DEGREE								
Married W. Child	9,603	100.0	6,977	72.7	2,303	24.0	323	3.4
Married No Child	3,429	100.0	2,834	82.6	510	14.8	85	2.5
Not Married W. Child	2,859	100.0	2,399	83.9	385	13.5	75	2.6
Not Married No Child	4,025	100.0	3,420	85.0	508	12.6	97	2.4

(continued)

Table 4.8 (continued)

BACCALAUREATE	TOTAL		ACTIVITY STATUS					
			Full-Time		Part-Time		Per Diem	
	Number	Percent	Number	Percent	Number	Percent	Number	Percent
Married W. Child	1,864	100.0	1,380	74.0	430	23.1	54	2.9
Married No Child	2,177	100.0	1,910	87.7	221	10.2	46	2.1
Not Married W. Child	659	100.0	569	86.3	74	11.3	16	2.4
Not Married No Child	4,311	100.0	3,929	91.1	311	7.2	71	1.6

Table 4.9 Mean Full-Time Salaries of Newly Licensed Nurses by Region and State of Employment, and Program Type, 1994

	TOTAL		Diploma		Associate Degree		Baccalaureate	
	Mean Salary	Standard Deviation	Mean Salary	Standard Deviation	Mean Salary	Standard Deviation	Mean Salary	Standard Deviation
UNITED STATES	29,384	5,934	30,189	5,684	29,027	5,944	29,890	5,924
NEW ENGLAND								
REGION TOTAL	31,739	5,704	33,127	5,040	30,926	5,846	32,308	5,583
Connecticut	35,008	5,099	34,868	4,043	35,207	5,568	34,879	5,155
Maine	27,416	4,310			27,167	4,759	27,802	3,502
Massachusetts	31,847	5,364	32,238	5,262	31,068	5,287	32,709	5,374
New Hampshire	27,811	7,863	25,475	6,086	25,651	7,405	30,192	8,469
Rhode Island	30,531	4,665	31,567	3,179	30,063	4,970	31,031	4,411
Vermont	26,745	3,705			26,601	3,565	27,128	4,199
MIDDLE ATLANTIC								
REGION TOTAL	33,183	7,153	31,977	5,863	32,778	7,315	34,780	7,389
New Jersey	36,027	4,977	35,832	4,307	35,437	4,857	37,123	5,500
New York	34,886	8,656	34,158	8,043	33,688	8,518	38,300	8,272
Pennsylvania	30,489	5,436	30,125	5,023	30,226	5,550	31,212	5,592

PROGRAM TYPE

(continued)

Table 4.9 (continued)

	TOTAL		Diploma		PROGRAM TYPE Associate Degree		Baccalaureate	
	Mean Salary	Standard Deviation	Mean Salary	Standard Deviation	Mean Salary	Standard Deviation	Mean Salary	Standard Deviation
EAST NORTH CENTRAL								
REGION TOTAL	28,638	4,861	33,127	5,040	30,926	5,846	29,354	5,583
Illinois	28,108	5,211	27,072	5,288	27,617	5,340	29,285	4,734
Indiana	27,849	4,803	27,146	5,378	27,598	5,015	28,378	4,297
Michigan	30,209	5,059	31,201	4,881	29,842	5,146	30,682	4,883
Ohio	28,988	4,337	29,207	4,347	28,281	4,454	29,989	3,922
Wisconsin	27,451	4,315	27,516	4,579	27,237	4,949	27,677	3,460
WEST NORTH CENTRAL								
REGION TOTAL	26,033	5,008	25,272	3,950	25,595	5,185	26,839	4,856
Iowa	24,192	4,919	23,750	4,415	23,837	4,875	25,971	5,180
Kansas	26,271	5,321	22,415	4,345	25,548	5,240	27,485	5,223
Minnesota	27,624	5,218			27,278	5,473	28,196	4,725
Missouri	26,660	4,702	26,168	3,492	26,135	4,992	27,710	4,685
Nebraska	25,126	4,418	25,830	2,498	25,031	4,352	25,137	4,576
North Dakota	24,731	3,443			24,112	4,176	24,781	3,406
South Dakota	24,252	4,211	21,950		24,020	4,438	24,811	3,724

(continued)

Table 4.9 (continued)

	TOTAL		Diploma		Associate Degree		Baccalaureate	
	Mean Salary	Standard Deviation	Mean Salary	Standard Deviation	Mean Salary	Standard Deviation	Mean Salary	Standard Deviation
SOUTH ATLANTIC								
REGION TOTAL	28,826	4,431	28,804	4,373	28,705	4,545	29,128	4,137
Delaware	32,098	5,585	29,670	822	32,061	5,752	32,584	5,591
District of Columbia	31,194	1,927	0	0	30,419	2,024	31,551	1,851
Florida	28,575	4,636	30,261	3,457	28,482	4,685	28,736	4,545
Georgia	28,787	4,349	30,000	0	28,595	4,539	29,280	3,786
Maryland	30,526	4,232	30,943	4,265	30,644	4,567	30,238	3,642
North Carolina	29,228	4,013	29,487	3,955	29,170	4,135	29,300	3,717
South Carolina	28,905	4,411	24,500	3,536	28,735	4,539	29,408	4,036
Virginia	27,906	4,171	27,084	4,488	27,850	4,055	28,442	4,171
West Virginia	26,226	3,888	28,285	3,814	26,117	3,797	25,934	4,074
EAST SOUTH CENTRAL								
REGION TOTAL	27,454	4,728	27,685	4,769	27,407	4,850	27,556	4,369
Alabama	27,608	5,029	26,118	4,498	27,514	4,995	28,067	5,168
Kentucky	27,065	4,366	0	0	26,916	4,382	27,504	4,299
Mississippi	28,835	5,287	32,000	7,211	28,978	5,456	28,292	4,647
Tennessee	26,898	4,300	27,913	4,636	26,772	4,521	26,916	3,603

PROGRAM TYPE

(continued)

Table 4.9 (continued)

	TOTAL		Diploma		Associate Degree		Baccalaureate	
	Mean Salary	Standard Deviation	Mean Salary	Standard Deviation	Mean Salary	Standard Deviation	Mean Salary	Standard Deviation
WEST SOUTH CENTRAL								
REGION TOTAL	29,248	5,938	29,362	4,963	29,076	5,944	29,613	5,993
Arkansas	25,283	4,978	26,936	1,908	25,393	5,109	24,861	4,715
Louisiana	32,926	6,660	0	0	32,808	6,825	33,051	6,490
Oklahoma	26,656	4,789	0	0	26,540	4,776	26,879	4,822
Texas	29,635	5,399	29,540	5,076	29,648	5,514	29,614	5,138
MOUNTAIN								
REGION TOTAL	26,651	4,658	27,120	5,770	26,572	4,589	26,807	4,798
Arizona	26,943	4,381	27,120	5,770	27,071	4,421	26,595	4,291
Colorado	27,160	4,597	0	0	27,304	4,768	27,016	4,431
Idaho	27,165	4,433	0	0	27,088	4,244	27,385	5,011
Montana	24,731	4,785	0	0	24,275	4,030	25,301	5,603
Nevada	28,767	4,478	0	0	28,150	4,344	29,433	4,584
New Mexico	27,558	4,760	0	0	27,885	4,916	26,313	3,941
Utah	25,954	4,706	0	0	25,731	4,186	26,633	6,025
Wyoming	23,978	3,959	0	0	23,812	3,890	24,532	4,209

PROGRAM TYPE

(continued)

Table 4.9 (continued)

	PROGRAM TYPE							
	TOTAL		Diploma		Associate Degree		Baccalaureate	
	Mean Salary	Standard Deviation	Mean Salary	Standard Deviation	Mean Salary	Standard Deviation	Mean Salary	Standard Deviation
PACIFIC								
REGION TOTAL	31,801	6,783	37,049	3,896	31,765	6,824	31,453	6,705
Alaska	31,765	4,423	0	0	33,183	4,851	30,703	4,063
California	33,380	6,834	37,049	3,896	33,262	6,821	33,175	7,061
Hawaii	30,486	8,449	0	0	36,000	0	29,567	8,864
Oregon	27,750	5,598	0	0	26,813	5,694	29,035	5,224
Washington	29,577	5,547	0	0	29,850	5,631	28,829	5,268

Table 4.10 Mean Part-Time Salaries of Newly Licensed Nurses by Region and State of Employment, and Program Type, 1994

	TOTAL		Diploma		Associate Degree		Baccalaureate	
	Mean Salary	Standard Deviation	Mean Salary	Standard Deviation	Mean Salary	Standard Deviation	Mean Salary	Standard Deviation
UNITED STATES	20,765	6,715	21,050	6,484	20,365	6,620	22,044	6,976
NEW ENGLAND								
REGION TOTAL	23,526	6,565	26,569	6,594	22,812	6,354	24,086	6,727
Connecticut	25,914	6,781	27,725	6,795	23,451	5,709	27,825	7,347
Maine	19,575	4,840	0	0	19,454	5,391	19,787	3,842
Massachusetts	23,669	6,571	25,610	6,315	23,312	6,615	23,860	6,509
New Hampshire	19,482	9,114	0	0	19,482	9,114	0	0
Rhode Island	24,520	5,858	26,544	8,164	23,878	5,393	25,450	6,480
Vermont	22,058	5,728	0	0	22,343	5,775	17,500	2,121
MIDDLE ATLANTIC								
REGION TOTAL	20,889	7,037	20,898	6,475	20,476	6,909	23,102	7,987
New Jersey	23,373	7,089	24,310	4,728	23,078	7,329	24,175	8,173
New York	20,831	7,190	22,366	7,410	20,465	7,021	23,305	8,171
Pennsylvania	20,194	6,743	20,106	6,389	19,476	6,347	22,798	7,962

PROGRAM TYPE

(continued)

Table 4.10 (continued)

	TOTAL		Diploma		PROGRAM TYPE Associate Degree		Baccalaureate	
	Mean Salary	Standard Deviation	Mean Salary	Standard Deviation	Mean Salary	Standard Deviation	Mean Salary	Standard Deviation
EAST NORTH CENTRAL								
REGION TOTAL	20,106	6,004	20,286	6,146	19,652	5,826	21,971	6,347
Illinois	19,650	6,629	16,746	6,016	19,231	6,289	22,980	7,763
Indiana	18,893	5,452	16,365	3,699	18,276	5,184	21,665	5,868
Michigan	21,854	6,640	23,914	6,528	21,197	6,445	24,044	7,075
Ohio	19,821	5,423	20,085	5,656	19,365	5,253	21,532	5,622
Wisconsin	20,041	5,415	22,500	8,226	19,910	5,403	20,270	5,291
WEST NORTH CENTRAL								
REGION TOTAL	18,816	5,536	18,398	4,636	18,629	5,589	19,426	5,719
Iowa	17,298	4,686	17,988	4,996	16,982	4,537	17,854	5,070
Kansas	19,082	6,008	19,667	2,517	19,468	6,352	18,380	5,978
Minnesota	19,722	5,789	0	0	19,216	5,804	21,015	5,581
Missouri	18,678	5,674	18,369	4,535	19,393	6,338	14,974	3,510
Nebraska	19,327	5,792	21,733	3,523	17,848	5,036	20,903	6,691
North Dakota	16,564	3,895	0	0	16,860	2,630	16,546	3,988
South Dakota	19,200	5,068	0	0	18,044	4,036	21,280	6,145

(continued)

Table 4.10 (continued)

| | PROGRAM TYPE | | | | | | | |
| | TOTAL | | Diploma | | Associate Degree | | Baccalaureate | |
	Mean Salary	Standard Deviation	Mean Salary	Standard Deviation	Mean Salary	Standard Deviation	Mean Salary	Standard Deviation
SOUTH ATLANTIC								
REGION TOTAL	20,234	6,040	21,600	6,027	20,030	6,052	20,610	5,992
Delaware	21,238	5,270	0	0	20,872	5,296	26,000	0
District of Columbia	28,352	498	0	0	28,352	498	0	0
Florida	21,033	6,776	30,000	0	20,660	7,236	21,691	4,935
Georgia	20,380	5,655	0	0	20,430	5,804	20,240	5,454
Maryland	21,176	5,005	26,200	5,374	21,174	5,106	19,755	3,813
North Carolina	18,981	6,000	18,817	4,175	18,796	6,094	20,117	6,963
South Carolina	21,564	5,507	0	0	22,074	5,475	19,730	5,830
Virginia	19,339	6,264	21,096	6,413	18,677	5,780	20,483	8,156
West Virginia	18,973	5,967	21,500	2,121	18,756	5,870	18,500	12,021
EAST SOUTH CENTRAL								
REGION TOTAL	20,031	6,529	19,042	6,735	18,997	6,188	23,047	6,657
Alabama	21,773	8,084	0	0	19,186	6,862	24,189	8,603
Kentucky	20,417	6,058	23,040	0	19,538	5,927	23,054	6,049
Mississippi	21,760	7,171	0	0	21,488	8,267	22,360	4,618
Tennessee	17,887	5,399	18,043	7,336	17,563	5,479	20,289	2,946

(continued)

Table 4.10 (continued)

	PROGRAM TYPE							
	TOTAL		Diploma		Associate Degree		Baccalaureate	
	Mean Salary	Standard Deviation	Mean Salary	Standard Deviation	Mean Salary	Standard Deviation	Mean Salary	Standard Deviation
PACIFIC								
REGION TOTAL	23,894	8,278	22,880	10,177	23,676	8,414	24,530	7,866
Alaska	24,296	5,791	0	0	22,699	964	25,493	7,873
California	26,484	8,641	22,507	12,431	26,701	8,855	26,035	7,941
Hawaii	0	0	0	0	0	0	0	0
Oregon	20,543	6,357	0	0	19,966	5,701	22,653	8,134
Washington	20,276	6,418	24,000	0	19,435	6,089	22,184	6,925

5

Survey of Newly Licensed Practical/ Vocational Nurses

Licensed practical/vocational nurses (LPN/LVNs), individuals who hold licenses to provide direct patient care under nursing supervision, were surveyed for the first time in 1994 by the NLN to collect data useful in (a) making informed decisions regarding the supply and demand for LPN/LVNs in the health care system and (b) helping educators prepare them appropriately in a changing health care system.

We have included in this book information from the results of the survey of newly licensed practical/vocational nurses. There is a significant number of these health care workers; an estimated 555,000 LPN/LVNs were employed in the United States as of December 1991.[2] Although the National Council of State Boards of Nursing routinely performs job analysis studies on LPN/LVNs, the NLN survey collected additional data in the areas of employment and educational characteristics.

METHODOLOGY

The purpose of this study was to collect information regarding the demographics, education, employment status, and

Note: References appear on p. 119.

intention of becoming a registered nurse of newly licensed PN/VNs in the United States.

The study used a different methodology from the survey of newly licensed nurses; a sample of the newly licensed PN/VNs were selected from those who had successfully completed their licensing examinations in October 1993. A stratified random sample was selected based on jurisdiction of licensure, and permission was sought from individual states to use their data tapes containing the names and addresses of newly licensed PN/VNs.

The survey tool contained 21 questions covering (a) demographic characteristics, (b) employment status, (c) perception of education, and (d) intention of becoming a registered nurse. Surveys were mailed to the sample cohort of newly licensed PN/VNs with a cover letter explaining the study.

RESULTS

Although not an extensive study, this survey yielded interesting information concerning the group of new LPN/LVNs and their impact on the future of the nursing workforce.

Demographic data. From the 1,704 respondents, the average age was 34.4 years. One hundred five (6.1%) of the respondents were over the age of 50. More than half of the respondents were between the ages of 26 and 41 (Table 5.2), and most were married (60.9%) (Figure 5.2), but 35.6 percent had no children at home (Figure 5.3). Many (36.6%) had children older than six years.

Employment status. More than half (53.0%) were employed in nursing and not seeking another job (Table 5.5). Of the 25 percent of all respondents who were employed in nursing but seeking other jobs, most (98.2%) were seeking jobs in nursing. Almost 22 percent were not employed in nursing; of those, 33.7 percent were not employed in nursing but seeking jobs in nursing, and 60.9 percent were not employed at all.

When asked why they were not employed in nursing, the most common response of the 368 respondents was continuing education (Figure 5.6). Many either could not find jobs (18.7%) or could not find the jobs they desired (7.1%).

Most (85.2%) of the employed respondents were still working at their first job (Table 5.3a). Thirty six (2.6%) respondents, however, were already working at their third (or more) job since receiving the license. Many (43.1%) of those employed found jobs before graduation (Table 5.3b). Most (69.9%) had found jobs by one month after graduation, although it took 3.3 percent more than six months. The two most common methods of finding a job were seeking employment at the clinical sites where their training took place (28.9%) and word of mouth (26.6%).

Many chose their jobs because of salary and benefits (37.9%) and/or because the jobs were in their desired specialty areas (28.4%) (Table 5.4). Few (6.6%) chose their jobs because of tuition reimbursement, which is surprising, given the numbers of respondents returning to school.

General duty nursing was overwhelmingly the most common type of position these respondents held (Figure 5.8). More than 10 percent held head nurse or assistant head nurse positions. The mean annual salary of all respondents was $17,788 (Figure 5.9). Most (70.8%) were not represented by a union, although almost 24 percent did not know if they were (Figure 5.16).

Perception of education. Respondents were asked to rate their clinical and classroom experiences. Most rated their classroom (61.0%) and clinical (60.4%) experiences as "very good" or "excellent" (Figure 5.5). Classroom experiences were rated slightly higher than clinical experiences.

Intention of becoming an RN. Most (83.0%) newly licensed PN/VNs planned to become registered nurses, and many (33.7%) were enrolled in nursing school at the time of the survey (Figures 5.12, 5.13). Another 51.6 percent planned to begin taking courses within one to three years.

Summary

Newly licensed PN/VNs were older than their nursing counterparts. Unlike the newly licensed nurses, they were able to
find jobs, including managerial positions. They rated their
educational experiences as adequate, and most intended to
continue with their education to become registered nurses.

The minority status of all students enrolled in PN/VN programs in 1992 (Figure 5.15), as well as the numbers of men
enrolled (Figure 5.14), has been determined in NLN's annual
survey, making some generalization possible.[3] It is evident
that men and minorities are underrepresented in this field.

Note: References appear on p. 119.

Figure 5.1 Sample Survey of New LPN/LVNs

EMPLOYMENT OF NEWLY LICENSED LPN/LVNS

1. Year of graduation: **19**☐☐ ← Write the year in the boxes.

   Then fill in the matching oval below each box.

2. Did you attend nursing school
   ① Full time?   ① Part time?

3. Did you work as a nurse's aide or an attendant before starting your LPN/LVN education?
   ① Yes   ② No

   3a. If yes, how long did you work as an aide or attendant before becoming an LPN/LVN?
   ① Never
   ① Less than 1 year
   ① 1-3 years
   ① 3-5 years
   ① Over 5 years

4. Mark **one** statement that most nearly corresponds to your most recent job-hunting experiences in nursing.
   ① Many jobs were available
   ① A fair number of jobs were available
   ① Very few jobs were available
   ① Can't say - took job at clinical site or previous employer
   ① Can't say - voluntarily unemployed

Complete either Question 5, 6 or 7 to best describe your current employment situation.

5. ○ I am employed in nursing - not seeking another job → Continue to Question 8.

6. I am employed in nursing -
   ○ but seeking other job in nursing ⎤ Continue to
   ○ but seeking other job **not** in nursing ⎦ Question 8.

7. ○ I am employed, **not** in nursing, but am seeking a job in nursing
   ○ I am employed, **not** in nursing, and am **not** seeking a job in nursing
   ○ I am presently not employed

7a. Main reason why not employed in nursing (mark only one):
   ① No jobs
   ① Jobs available, but couldn't find what I wanted
   ① Continuing my education
   ① Family responsibilities
   ① Have relocated
   ① Don't want to practice nursing
   ① Other (specify: _____)

7b. How long have you been actively seeking a nursing job?
   ① One month or less ⎤
   ① Two to three months
   ① Four to six months ⎬ → Skip to Question 16.
   ① Over six months
   ① Not seeking a job ⎦

8. Since receiving your PN/VN license, is this your -
   ① 1st?
   ② 2nd?
   ③ 3rd or more job in nursing?

9. How long after graduation did it take you to find your first job in nursing? (Mark **one**)
   ① Found the job before graduation
   ① One month or less
   ① Two to three months
   ① Four to six months
   ① Over six months

10. How did you find out about your current job? (Mark **one**)
   ① Classified ad in newspaper/journal
   ① Word-of-mouth
   ① Faculty recommendation
   ① Clinical site for nursing school/previous employer
   ① On-site recruiter
   ① Employment agency
   ① Other (specify: _____)

11. Mark the **two** main reasons for choosing your current position.
   ① Amount of vacation/holidays
   ② Housing
   ③ Health insurance
   ④ Tuition reimbursement
   ⑤ Salary/benefits
   ⑥ Promotional opportunities
   ⑦ Desired this specialization
   ⑧ Other (specify: _____)

Continue on back

◧■○■○■■○■■■○○○○○○○○○○○○   **5994**
DO NOT WRITE IN THIS SHADED AREA

Figure 5.1 (continued)

12. Type of position:
- ⊙ General duty/staff
- ⊙ Head nurse/assistant
- ⊙ Private duty
- ⊙ Other (specify: _____)

13. Please specify the annual earnings from your <u>primary</u> nursing position before tax deductions. Do NOT include overtime.

← Write the amount in the boxes.

← Then fill in the matching oval below each box.

14. How well did your classroom and clinical experiences prepare you for your current job?

a. Classroom
- ⊙ Excellent
- ⊙ Very good
- ⊙ Good
- ⊙ Fair
- ⊙ Poor

b. Clinical
- ⊙ Excellent
- ⊙ Very good
- ⊙ Good
- ⊙ Fair
- ⊙ Poor

15. Are you represented by a labor association that has a contract for collective bargaining?
- ⊙ Yes
- ⊙ No
- ⊙ Don't know

16. Do you plan to become an RN?
- ⊙ Yes   ⊙ No

16a. If yes, when? (Mark <u>one</u>)
- ⊙ I am currently taking courses
- ⊙ Within 1-2 years
- ⊙ Within 2-3 years
- ⊙ Within 4-5 years
- ⊙ More than 5 years

17. Year of birth:

← Write the year in the boxes.

← Then fill in the matching oval below each box.

18. Marital status:
- ⊙ Never married
- ⊙ Married
- ⊙ Separated/Divorced
- ⊙ Widowed

19. Children living at home most of the time are: (Mark <u>one</u>)
- ⊙ No children at home
- ⊙ All less than 6 years old
- ⊙ All 6 years or older
- ⊙ Both younger and older than 6 years

20. What is the zip code of your home address?

← Write the zip code in the boxes.

← Then fill in the matching oval below each box.

21. What is the zip code of your current place of employment?

← Write the zip code in the boxes.

← Then fill in the matching oval below each box.

The National League for Nursing thanks you for your participation in this survey.

Figure 5.2 Marital Status of Newly Licensed PN/VNs, 1994

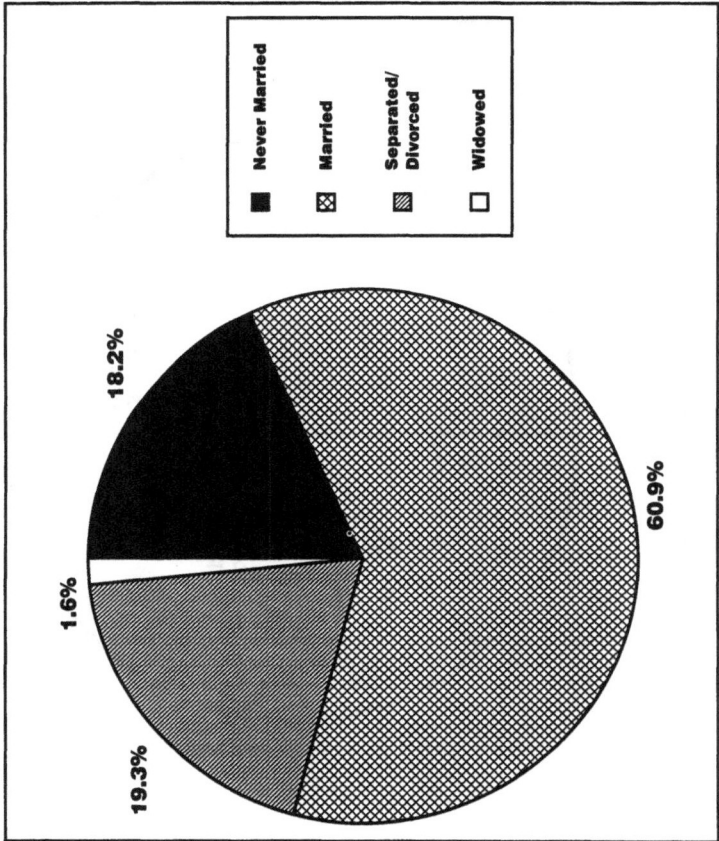

Never Married
Married
Separated/Divorced
Widowed

18.2%
60.9%
1.6%
19.3%

Figure 5.3   Presence of Children in the Homes of Newly Licensed PN/VNs, 1994

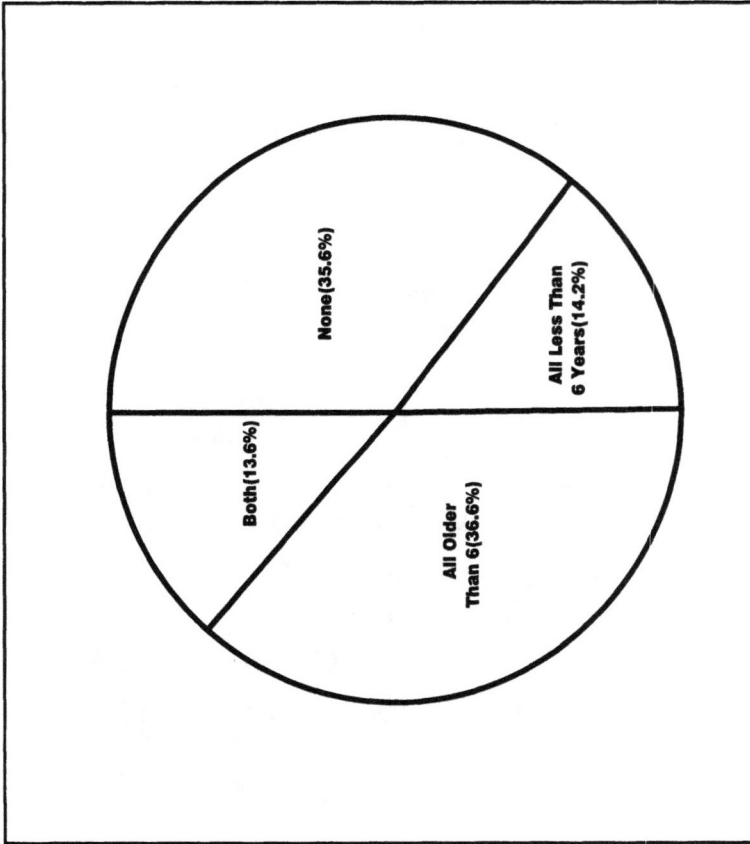

Figure 5.4   Nursing School Attendance of Newly Licensed PN/VNs, 1994

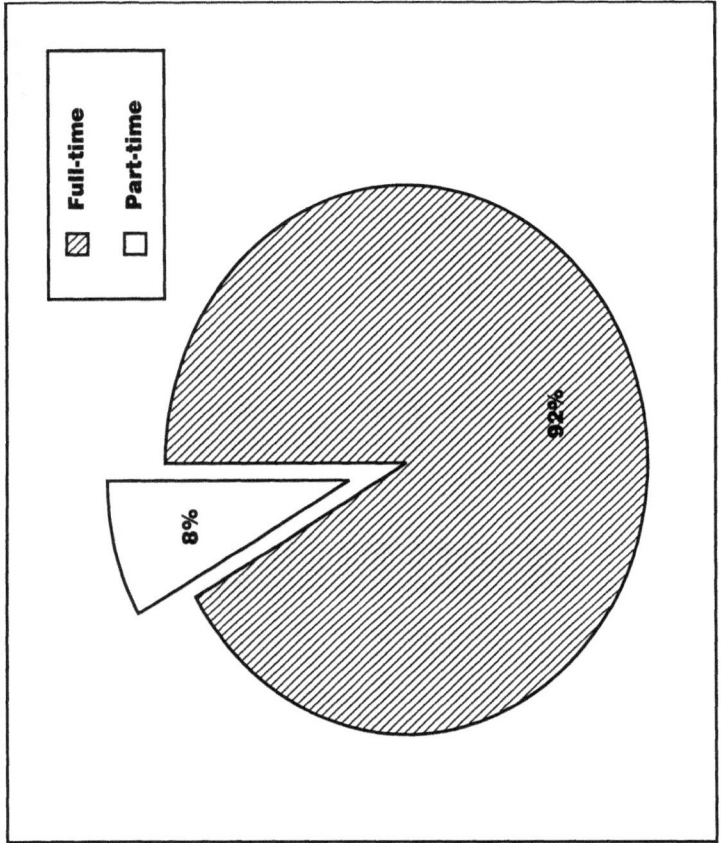

Legend:
- Full-time
- Part-time

92%

8%

Figure 5.5 Newly Licensed PN/VNs Rating of Classroom and Clinical Experience, 1994

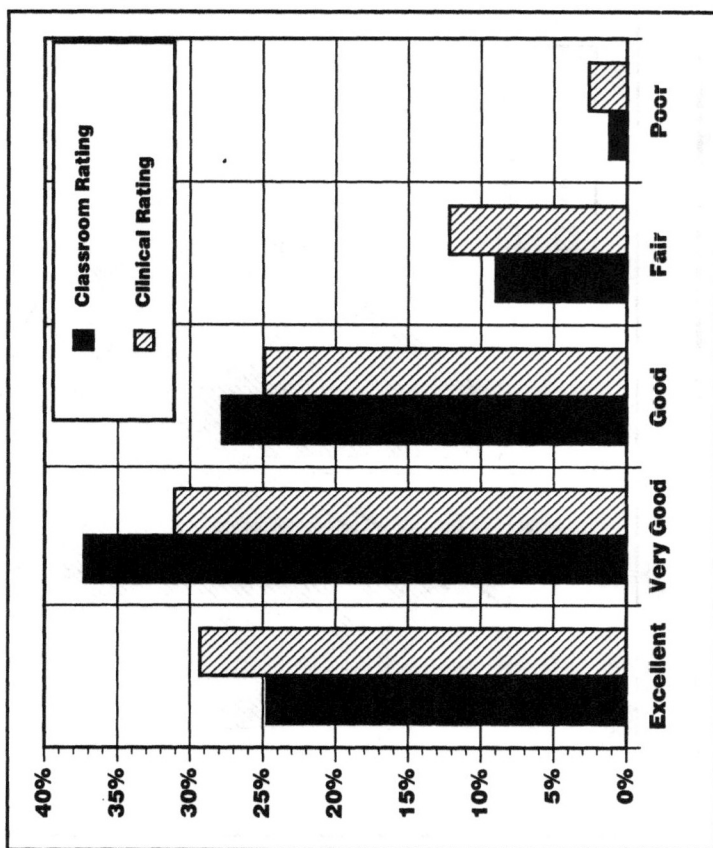

Figure 5.6   Main Reason Why Newly Licensed PN/VNs Were Not Employed in Nursing, 1994

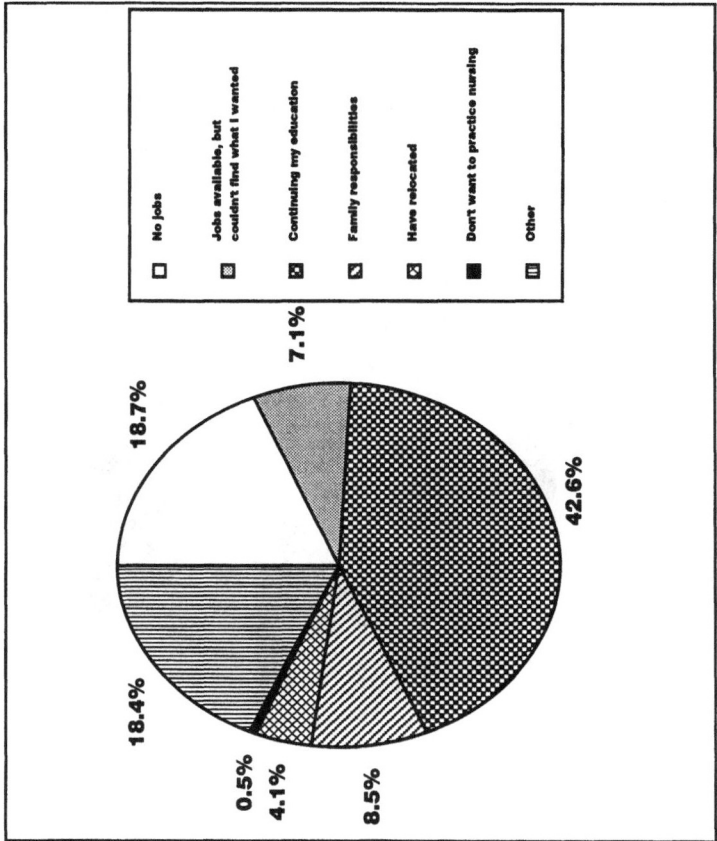

Legend:
- ☐ No jobs
- ▨ Jobs available, but couldn't find what I wanted
- ▧ Continuing my education
- ▨ Family responsibilities
- ▨ Have relocated
- ■ Don't want to practice nursing
- ▦ Other

Percentages shown: 18.7%, 7.1%, 42.6%, 8.5%, 4.1%, 0.5%, 18.4%

Figure 5.7   Perception of Job Availability of Newly Licensed PN/VNs, 1994

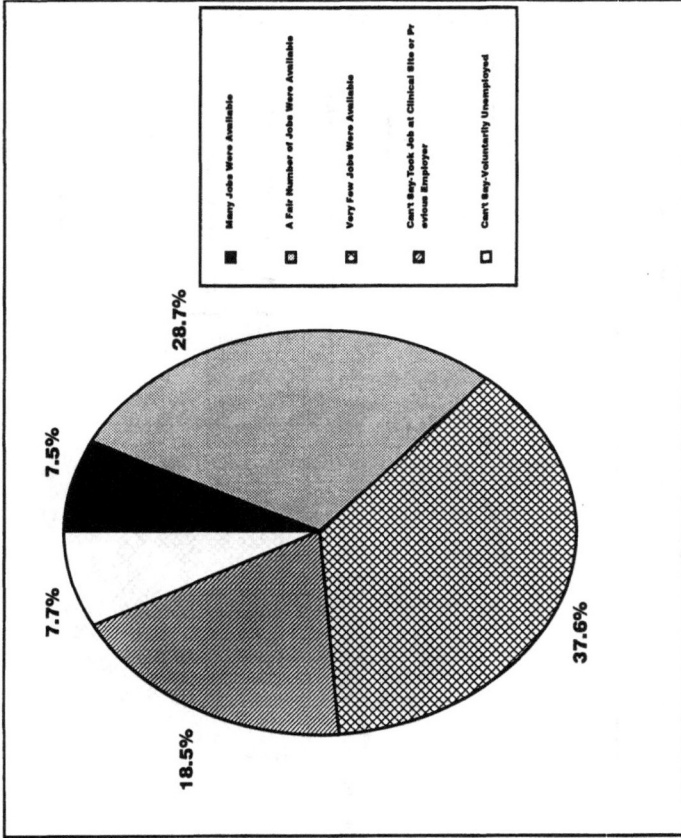

Legend:
- ■ Many Jobs Were Available
- ▨ A Fair Number of Jobs Were Available
- ▨ Very Few Jobs Were Available
- ▨ Can't Say-Took Job at Clinical Site or Previous Employer
- □ Can't Say-Voluntarily Unemployed

28.7%
7.5%
7.7%
18.5%
37.6%

Figure 5.8   Type of Positions Held by Newly Licensed PN/VNs, 1994

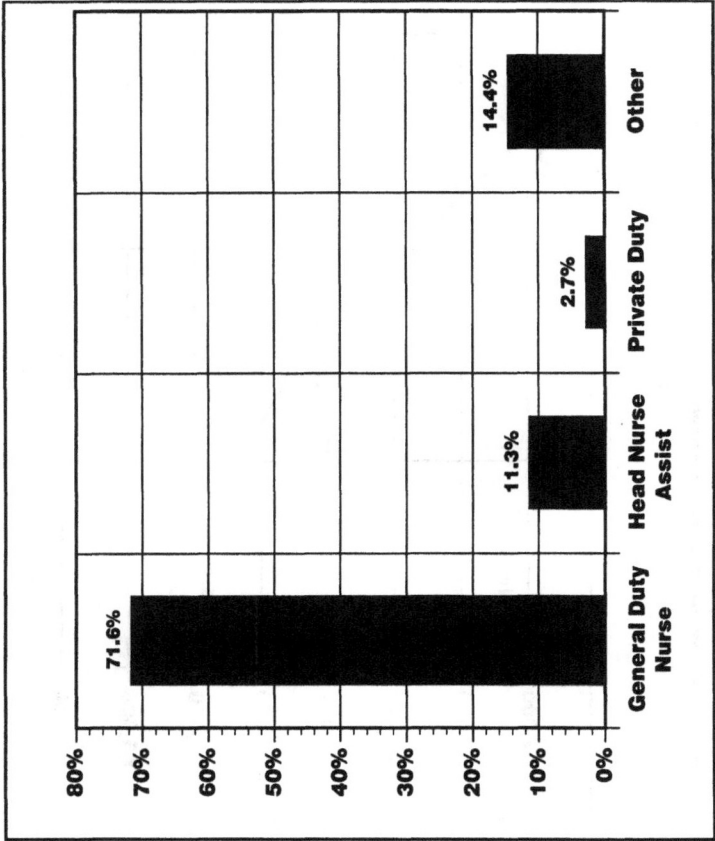

Figure 5.9   Mean Salary of Newly Licensed PN/VNs, 1994

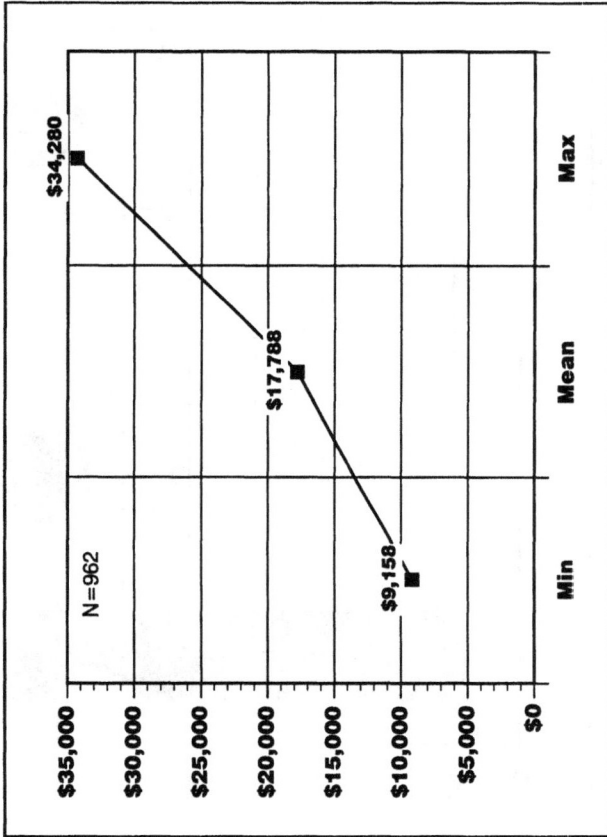

Figure 5.10 Newly Licensed PN/VNs Who Had Prior Experience as a Nurse's Aide

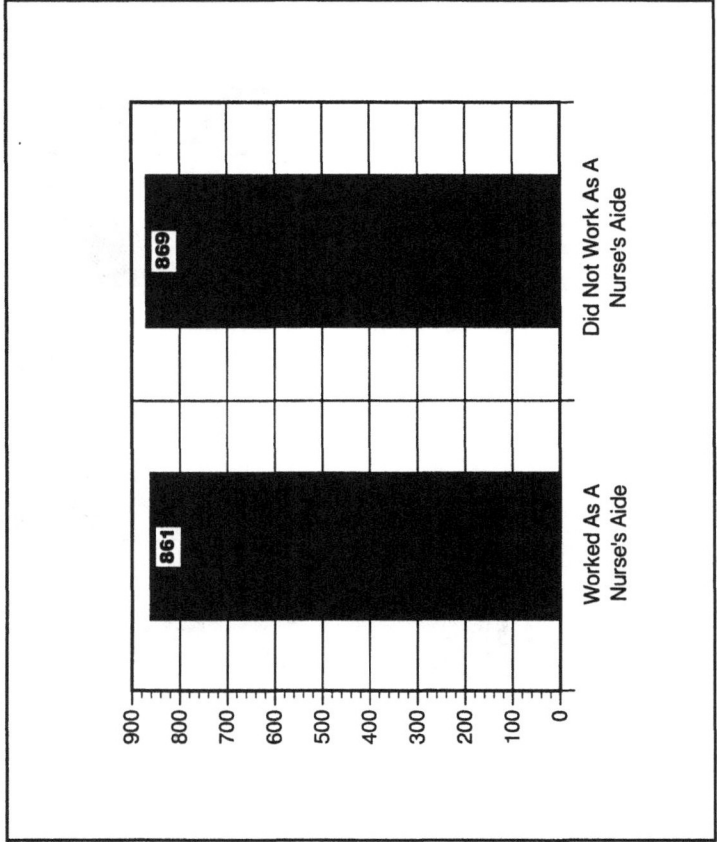

Figure 5.11 Length of Time Newly Licensed PN/VNs Worked as Nurse's Aide, 1994

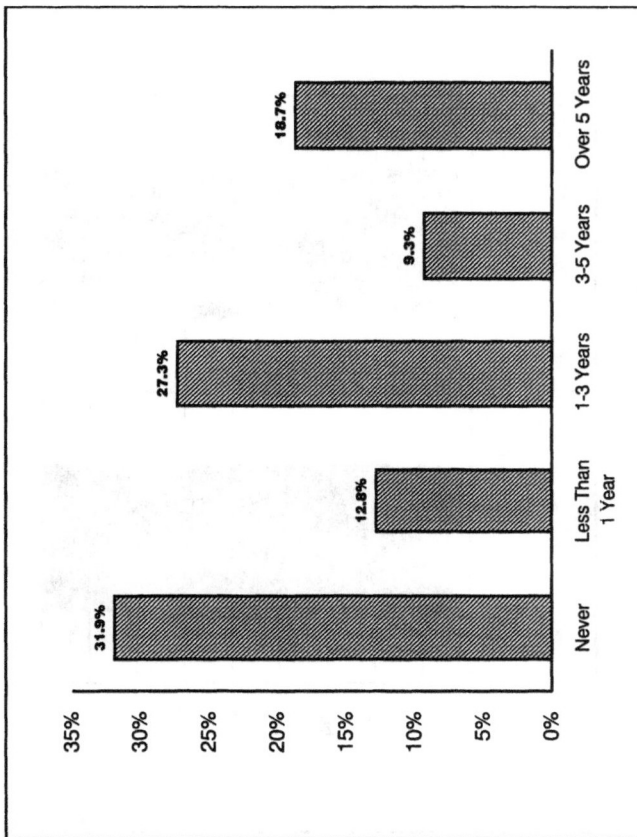

Category	Percentage
Never	31.9%
Less Than 1 Year	12.8%
1-3 Years	27.3%
3-5 Years	9.3%
Over 5 Years	18.7%

Figure 5.12 Percentage of Newly Licensed PN/VNs *Who* Plan to Become
Registered Nurses, 1994

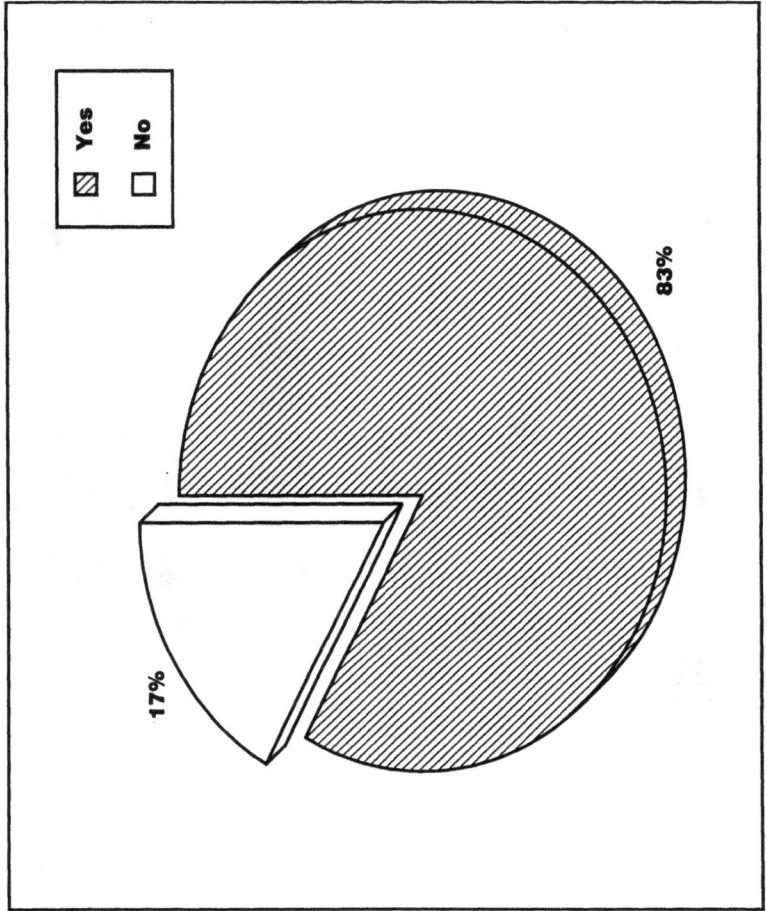

Figure 5.13 When Newly Licensed PN/VNs Plan to Become Registered Nurses

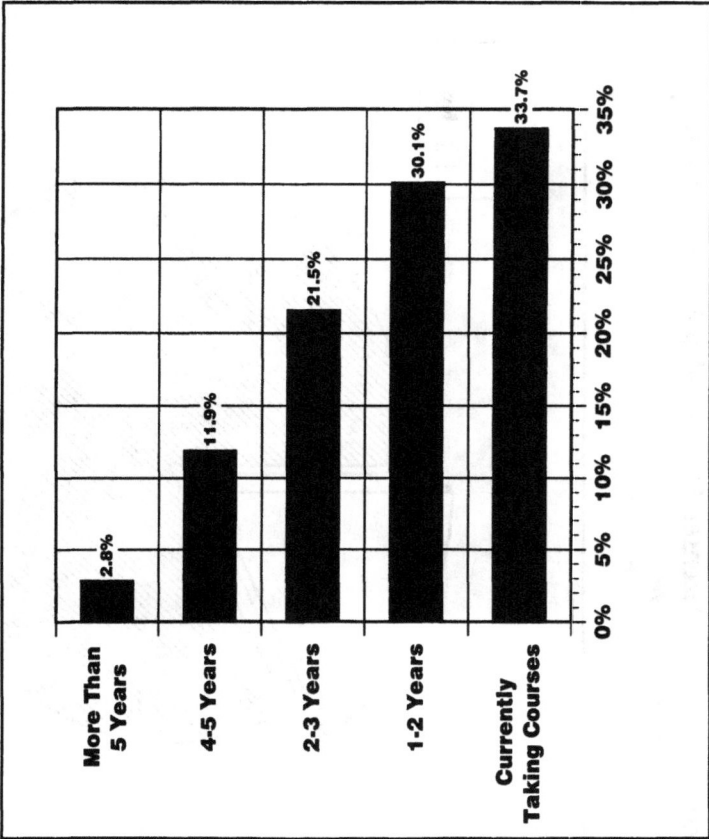

Figure 5.14 Percentage of Men in LPN/LVN Programs, 1992, 1994

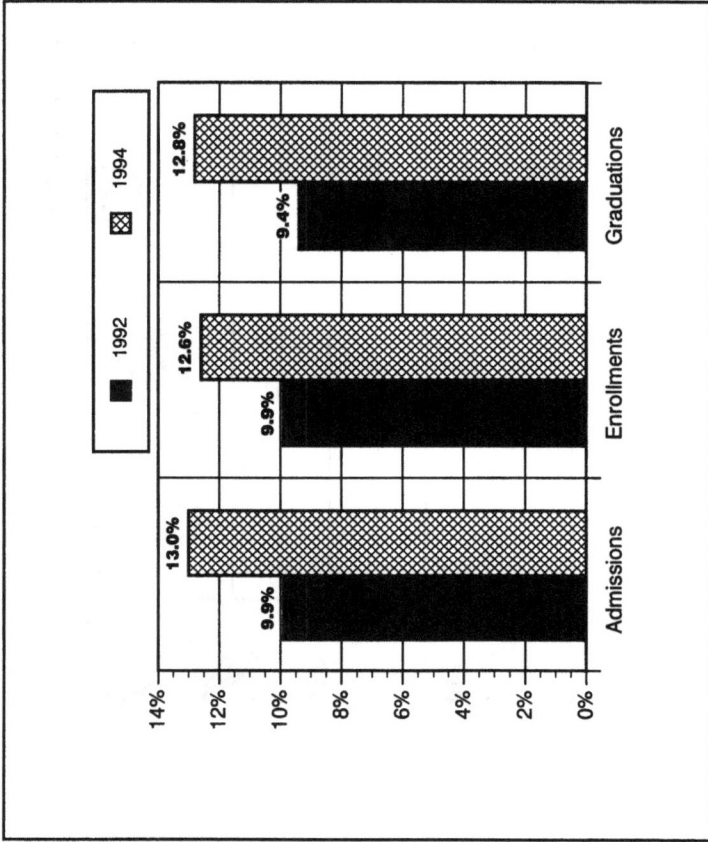

■ 1992   ▨ 1994

	1992	1994
Admissions	9.9%	13.0%
Enrollments	9.9%	12.6%
Graduations	9.4%	12.8%

Source: *Nursing DataSource 1995, Volume III.*

Figure 5.15 Percentage of Minorities Enrolled in LPN/LVN Programs, 1992, 1994

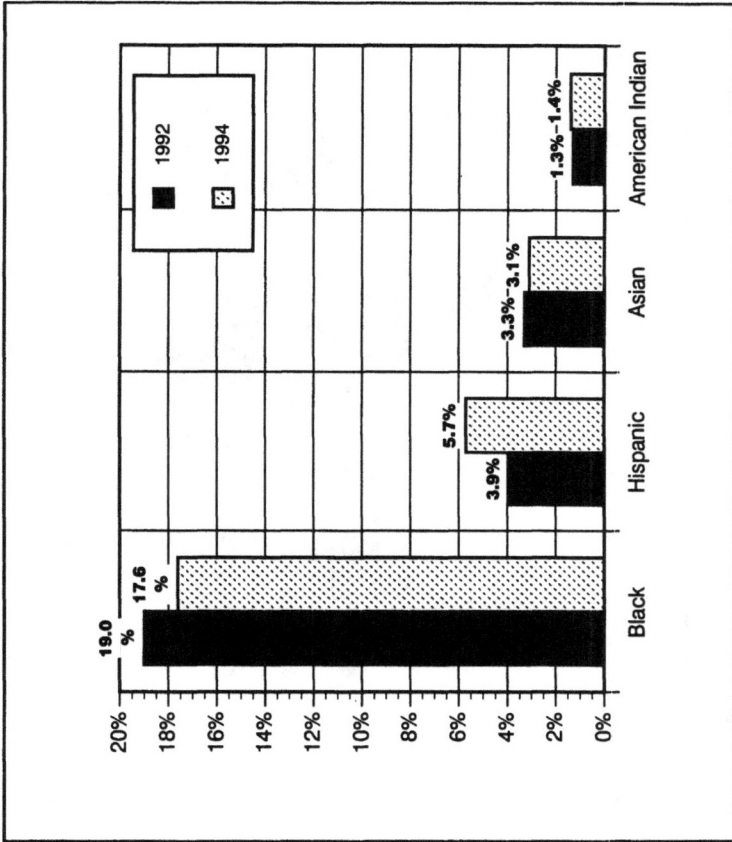

■ 1992
▨ 1994

	Black	Hispanic	Asian	American Indian

19.0% 17.6% (Black)
3.9% 5.7% (Hispanic)
3.3%–3.1% (Asian)
1.3%–1.4% (American Indian)

Source: *Nursing DataSource 1995, Volume III*

Figure 5.16 Percentage of Newly Licensed PN/VNs Represented by a Union

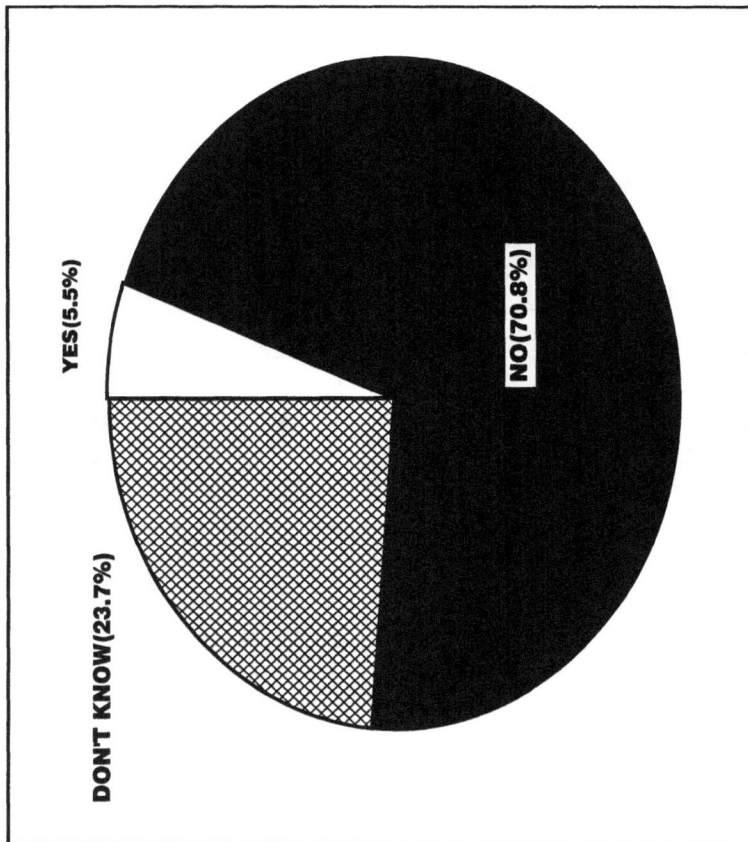

YES(5.5%)

DON'T KNOW(23.7%)

NO(70.8%)

Table 5.1 Trends in the Estimated Number of Graduations of Minority Students from LPN/LVN Programs: 1989–90 to 1993–94[1]

YEAR	BLACK		HISPANIC		ASIAN		AMERICAN INDIAN	
	Number	Percent	Number	Percent	Number	Percent	Number	Percent
ALL REGIONS								
1989-90	5,240	14.8	1,584	4.5	730	2.1	289	0.8
1990-91	5,421	14.2	1,720	4.5	956	2.5	260	0.7
1991-92	6,575	15.7	1,628	3.9	1,329	3.2	415	1.0
1992-93	7,785	17.4	2,298	5.1	1,115	2.5	363	0.8
1993-94	6,463	14.3	1,942	4.3	1,594	3.5	453	1.0
NORTH ATLANTIC								
1989-90	1,129	17.4	187	2.9	66	1.0	14	0.2
1990-91	1,324	18.5	156	2.2	80	1.1	8	0.1
1991-92	1,368	17.9	194	2.5	185	2.4	56	0.7
1992-93	1,839	21.2	295	3.4	113	1.3	24	0.3
1993-94	1,503	16.6	258	2.8	184	2.0	40	0.4
MIDWEST								
1989-90	987	10.8	78	0.8	63	0.7	53	0.6
1990-91	845	8.6	175	1.8	111	1.6	49	0.5
1991-92	1,161	10.9	188	1.8	170	1.6	79	0.7
1992-93	1,138	10.2	288	2.6	131	1.2	49	0.4
1993-94	1,037	9.2	216	1.9	252	2.2	85	0.7
SOUTH								
1989-90	2,582	18.1	707	5.0	99	0.7	152	1.1
1990-91	2,892	18.4	825	5.3	156	5.6	134	0.9
1991-92	3,314	19.0	659	3.8	252	1.4	149	0.8
1992-93	4,248	23.0	901	4.9	214	1.2	166	0.9
1993-94	3,176	17.0	954	5.1	546	2.9	258	1.4
WEST								
1989-90	542	9.8	612	11.0	502	9.0	70	1.3
1990-91	360	6.7	564	10.1	609	10.9	69	1.2
1991-92	732	11.8	587	9.4	722	11.6	131	2.1
1992-93	560	8.6	814	12.5	657	10.1	124	1.9
1993-94	747	12.3	514	8.5	612	10.1	70	1.2

[1] Excludes American Samoa, Guam, Puerto Rico, and the Virgin Islands.

Table 5.2   Mean Age of Newly Licensed PN/VNs, 1994

	TOTAL: 1704 MEAN: 34.4	
AGE	NUMBER	PERCENT
18–25	323	19.0
26–33	507	29.8
34–41	503	29.5
42-49	266	15.6
50–57	96	5.6
58–65	9	0.5

Table 5.3a Job Number of Newly Licensed PNs/VNs, 1994

	COUNT	PERCENT
1st Job	1179	85.2
2nd Job	168	12.1
3rd or More	36	2.6
Total	1383	100.0

**Table 5.3b Length of Time for Newly Licensed PN/VNs
to Find First Job**

	COUNT	PERCENT
Before Graduation	587	43.1
1 Month or Less	365	26.8
2–3 Months	243	17.8
4–6 Months	123	9.0
Over 6 Months	45	3.3
Total	1363	100.0

**Table 5.3c How Newly Licensed PN/VNs Found
Their Current Jobs, 1994**

	COUNT	PERCENT
Classified Ad	235	17.4
Word of Mouth	359	26.6
Faculty Recommendation	69	5.1
Clinical Site	389	28.9
On-Site Recruiter	40	3.0
Agency	21	1.6
Other	235	17.4
Total	1348	100.0

Table 5.4   Reasons Why Newly Licensed PN/VNs Chose Their Current Position

	Salary/Benefits		Promotion Opportunites	
	COUNT	PERCENT	COUNT	PERCENT
YES	671	37.9	146	8.2
NO	1099	62.1	1624	91.8
Total	1770	100.0	1770	100.0

	Health Insurance		Tuition Reimbursement	
	COUNT	PERCENT	COUNT	PERCENT
YES	210	11.9	116	6.6
NO	1560	88.1	1654	93.4
Total	1770	100.0	1770	100.0

	Amount of Vacation		Housing	
	COUNT	PERCENT	COUNT	PERCENT
YES	41	2.3	19	1.1
NO	1729	97.7	1751	98.9
Total	1770	100.0	1770	100.0

	Specialization		Other Reason	
	COUNT	PERCENT	COUNT	PERCENT
YES	503	28.4	524	29.6
NO	1267	71.6	1246	70.4
Total	1770	100.0	1770	100.0

Table 5.5   Current Employment Status of Newly Licensed PN/VNs, 1994

Employed in nursing— Not seeking another job	NUMBER	PERCENT
YES	938	53.0
NO	832	47.0
Employed in nursing	NUMBER	PERCENT
Seeking other job in nursing	436	98.2
Seeking other job *not* in nursing	8	1.8
Employed not in nursing	NUMBER	PERCENT
Employed, *not* in nursing, but seeking a job in nursing	124	33.7

Employed, *not* in nursing, and
  am *not* seeking a job
  in nursing
	20	5.4

Presently not employed	224	60.9

6

Newly Licensed Nurses– Final Thoughts

"I love my job." (Wyoming)

"The classified ads are deceiving—lots of RN positions—but not for new grads." (Ohio)

"Of the 65 people graduating BSN '93, 3 got jobs full-time in an area hospital. It's bad!"
(Washington)

"Nurses are expected to do too much in too little time and take care of too many patients—at least on my floor. They staff by numbers, not acuity level. It leads to too much stress and all patients get less time than they need." (Colorado)

The results from the 1994 survey reflect changes in recruitment of nursing students and the impact of the changing health care system on new graduates. There are patterns of change that are welcome, but there are also warning signs of less desirable trends. The comments included on survey forms and in attached letters indicated that nurses newly licensed in 1994 were dedicated, compassionate, and eager to be nurses. Common themes ran throughout their comments.

The first theme was that of a love for nursing. Even when the job situation was difficult, a love for the profession was evident: "I enjoy nursing; however, our floor is worked with a short staff on purpose to make money, so I feel that my patients do not get the attention and care that a hospitalized person should receive" (Georgia). Many comments reflected a concern for the quality of care patients received.

The second theme concerned the unwillingness of employers to hire new graduates. Even when jobs were available, criteria for hiring included one to two years of experience. As one respondent wrote, "How do you get experience if no one will hire you?" (Pennsylvania). Several commented that the only way to get a job was by knowing someone who had "pull."

The third theme, and the one that elicited the most frustration and anger, was the lack of jobs of any kind. Respondents from every geographical area reported a lack of job openings Some were able to find jobs that required a great deal of inconvenience: "I have to commute 1 ½ hours each way to my job. It was the only place I could find work..." (California). Many worked several part-time jobs.

> Conversely, those who had found employment felt overworked: The nursing profession is becoming very overworked in the hospital with much understaffing, loss of nursing assistants, and nurses being expected to do everyone's jobs, including transportation, nursing assistant, and respiratory care, with patient loads of between 7 to 9 patients to a nurse. (Florida)

These nurses are being given heavy workloads and cannot spend the time they feel is necessary with their patients. They noted that patient care is suffering.

It is interesting to note that there seemed to be too many newly licensed nurses for the positions available, but those employed found too few nurses for the workload. This raises questions such as how staffing decisions were made and is possibly a reflection of an emphasis on cost savings in a changing health care delivery system.

Several respondents commented on the treatment they received from other nurses. For example, one respondent wrote: "The most difficult part of being a new nurse is that older, more experienced nurses are not supportive or encouraging. Most have bad attitudes" (Missouri). Apparently, the age-old problem of nurses "eating their young" (quoted by another respondent) was still experienced by some of the newest nurses in 1994.

In summary, the survey of newly licensed nurses of 1994 yielded vital information to those concerned with the health care delivery workforce in the United States. Patterns of change were evident in the demographics, educational experiences, and employment status of this group. The feedback and the information they shared portend much about the future issues of nursing practice.

TABLE 6.1 Graduations from Basic RN Programs and Percentage Change from Previous Year, by Program Type, 1974-75 to 1993-94

| | PROGRAM TYPE | | | | | | | |
| | TOTAL | | Diploma | | Associate Degree | | Baccalaureate | |
ACADEMIC YEAR	Number	Percent	Number	Percent	Number	Percent	Number	Percent
1974-75	73,915	+10.2	21,562	+1.8	32,183	+11.3	20,170	+18.9
1975-76	77,065	+4.3	19,861	-7.9	34,625	+7.6	22,579	+11.9
1976-77	77,755	+0.9	18,014	-9.3	36,289	+4.8	23,452	+3.9
1977-78	77,874	+0.1	17,131	-4.9	36,556	+0.7	24,187	+3.1
1978-79	77,132	-1.0	15,820	-7.7	36,264	-0.8	25,048	+3.6
1979-80	75,523	-2.1	14,495	-8.4	36,034	-0.6	24,994	-0.2
1980-81	73,985	-2.0	12,903	-11.0	36,712	+1.9	24,370	-2.5
1981-82	74,052	+0.1	11,682	-9.5	38,289	+4.3	24,081	-1.2
1982-83	77,408	+4.5	11,704	+0.2	41,849	+9.3	23,855	-0.9
1983-84	80,312	+3.8	12,200	+4.2	44,394	+6.1	23,718	-0.6
1984-85	82,075	+2.2	11,892	-2.5	45,208	+1.8	24,975	+5.3
1985-86	77,027	-6.2	10,524	-11.5	41,333	-8.6	25,170	+0.8
1986-87	70,561	-8.4	8,272	-21.4	38,528	-6.8	23,761	-5.6
1987-88	64,839	-8.0	5,938	-28.2	37,397	-2.9	21,504	-9.5
1988-89	61,660	-4.9	4,826	-18.7	37,837	+1.2	18,997	-11.6
1989-90	66,088	+7.2	5,199	+7.7	42,318	+11.8	18,571	-2.2
1990-91	72,230	+9.3	6,172	+18.7	46,794	+10.6	19,264	+3.7
1991-92	80,839	+11.9	6,528	+5.8	52,896	+13.0	21,415	+11.2
1992-93	88,149	+9.0	6,937	+6.3	56,770	+7.3	24,442	+14.1
1993-94	94,870	+7.6	7,119	+2.6	58,839	+3.6	28,912	+18.3

REFERENCES

1. Rosenfeld, P., & Moses, E.B. (1988). Nursing supply and demand: An analysis of newspaper, journal, and newsletters. *Nursing & Health Care,* 9(5), 248–252.

2. 9th Report to Congress. Department of Health and Human Services. *Health Personnel in the United States.* (1993)

3. National League for Nursing Research. *Nursing DataSource III: Focus on Practical/Vocational Nursing, 1995.*

www.ingramcontent.com/pod-product-compliance
Lightning Source LLC
Chambersburg PA
CBHW070736220326
41598CB00024BA/3440